Acclaim for *Kara Mia*

*"Often a silver lining exists in clouds of darkness...Long QT syndrome is a very treatable disorder and the events can be prevented if the disease is recognized early...*Kara Mia *will educate and inform...Precious lives will be saved as a consequence of this effort."*

From the Foreword by G. Michael Vincent, M.D.,
Chairman, Department of Medicine, LDS Hospital,
Professor of Medicine, University of Utah

"Starting with a tale of a life-threatening illness told through the letters of Kara's teenage friends, I experienced the powerful interplay among optimistic kids, an insightful mom, and an emotionally available physician. Good Stuff!"

Susan B. Soule, LCSW, Project Coordinator
for Parents in Partnership

"Kara's story is an inspiration and should be read by anyone who has been touched by Long QT syndrome so they will know they are not alone."

Katie Roberts, SADS Foundation

"Kara Mia *is difficult to categorize. In one sense, it is a positive addition to the body of writing known as 'parent accounts' but it is more than that. It is also an important and informative contribution to public awareness about a silent health threat but it is more than that. It is an account of the subjective, tenuous practice of medicine and the degree to which this is an art as well as a science—but it is more than that, too. It offers insight into the workings of the physician—family relationship, as we readers witness how a professional, in caring for his child/patient, is drawn into caring about her and about her family.* **Kara Mia** *will find a unique and valuable place for itself; I feel privileged to have read it."*

Elaine H. Walizer, author of *Building the Healing Partnership: Parents, Professionals, and Children with Chronic Illnesses and Disabilities*

Kara Mia

*the story of sudden loss and slow recovery
in a teenager with Long QT syndrome*

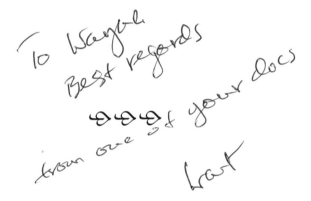

By Maryann Anglim & Walter Allan, M.D.

Seahorse Press
Bath, Maine

Grateful acknowledgment is made to the following for permission to reprint
previously published material: Excerpt from *bird by bird* by Anne Lamott,
copyright © 1994 by Anne Lamott, reprinted by permission of the author.
Excerpt from "Love Hurts" by writer Boudleaux Bryant © 1960 by Acuff-Rose
Publications, Inc. Renewed 1988 by House of Bryant Publications, P.O. Box
570, Gatlinburg, TN, USA, 37738. Excerpt from "Because You Loved Me,"
words and music by Diane Warren © 1996 Realsongs and Touchstone Pictures
Music & Songs, Inc. All rights reserved. Used by permission. Warner Bros.
Publications U.S. Inc., Miami, FL, 33014. Excerpt from "Fly" J.J. Goldman/Phil
Gladston, Les Editions JRG/CRB Music Publishing (SOCAN) administered by
Sony Music Publishing Canada. Copyright © 1996-All rights reserved on behalf
of Sony Music Publishing Canada/CRB Music Publishing adm. by Sony/ATV
Music Publishing LLC (ASCAP), 8 Music Sq. W., Nashville, TN, USA, 37203. All
rights reserved. Used by permission.

Some of the names of persons mentioned in this book have been changed to
protect their privacy.

Cataloging-in-Publication Data:
Anglim, Maryann (1949 -   ) and Walter Allan, M.D. (1943 -   )
Kara Mia: the story of sudden loss and slow recovery in a teenager with Long
QT syndrome / by Maryann Anglim and Walter Allan, M.D.
ISBN 0-9656501-0-3   Library of Congress Catalog Card Number: 97-91509

1. Heart-Diseases. 2. Long QT syndrome. I. Allan, Walter, M.D. II. Title.
616.1 1997

Cover art by Janice Wright.

Book design by Thomas Hillman Design.

Printed by McNaughton & Gunn, Inc., Saline, Michigan, on 50% recycled fiber
paper in the United States of America.

❧ ❧ ❧

Dedication

❧ ❧ ❧

The task of choosing to whom to dedicate this book was a daunting one. There were many deserving candidates. Should we dedicate it to Alan Douglass and David Hudson and their paramedic team? Those were the men who saved Kara's life on the track on April 7, 1995. Should we dedicate it to Dr. Rebecca Chagrasulis and the Bath Midcoast Hospital emergency room? Those were the people who sustained Kara's vital signs as she tottered between life and death that day. Should we dedicate it to the medical staff and employees of Maine Medical Center? Those were the people who lead Kara back to health as she recovered under their special guidance.

Should we dedicate *Kara Mia* to our friends and neighbors? These were the people who cleaned our house, fed us for four months, mowed our lawn and walked the dog. Should we dedicate it to my co-workers in the operating room? These were the people who gave me all the easy cases until my feet were firmly planted on the ground once again. Should we dedicate it to certain special friends who have been more angelic than human? These were the people who helped me give Kara her first bed bath (that would be you, Linda) or who literally held my hand through the first surgical case I did on my first day back to work (that would be you, John) or who gave Kara her weekly shampoo and manicure (that would be you, Paula) or despite an ankle broken while rescuing puppies, unfailingly had Kara to her house every Tuesday (that would be you, Joanna). Should we dedicate the book to our technical support staff? These were the people who read and reread our manuscript and generously offered us their computer expertise.

Dedication

Should we dedicate the book to my parents? They were the ones who heard the news of Kara's collapse at 4:00 p.m. in Chicago and were in Maine by 9:00 p.m. that night. Should we dedicate this book to our respective children, Ken, who is in graduate school at the University of Chicago, and Guerin, who is a sophomore at Providence College? We are proud of both of them. Should we dedicate this book to our respective spouses, Ann and Tom? They have been more than tolerant of our writing process in their quiet, calm, patient and funny ways. They have always had faith in us, stood beside us and trusted the importance of this book to us.

Even though all of these people are deserving of a dedication, there is one person who transcends all of them and that person is Kara. So, Kara, we dedicate this book to you. This book is a testament to your smiling hard work and this bittersweet story of love and modern medicine. You have taught us that miracles do happen.

❦ ❦ ❦

Table of Contents

❦ ❦ ❦

༄ ༄ ༄

❧ ❧ ❧

Foreword

❧ ❧ ❧

A hymn states, "When upon life's billows you are tempest tossed, when you are discouraged thinking all is lost, count your many blessings, name them one by one, and it will surprise you what the Lord has done." While *Kara Mia* is a tale of tragedy wrought by the Long QT syndrome, it is also a beautiful story of courage, strength, and faith, and the ability of the human spirit to rise above and grow from the challenges and hurdles which are placed into the lives of many of us.

Kara Mia's story is common in the Long QT syndrome—a completely unexpected cardiac arrest or sudden death, or unexplained loss of consciousness (syncope), in an apparently healthy young person. Once thought to be rare, the syndrome is now recognized as a common cause of these events. The disorder is due to mutations in genes which control the electrical activity of the heart. Affected persons are predisposed to a sudden onset, very fast and abnormal heart rhythm, which causes the syncope, cardiac arrest, or sudden cardiac death. These events typically occur during the preteen to teenage years; they can occur as early as the first days or weeks of life and infrequently even as late as the fourth or fifth decade. Some patients never have any symptoms, but still can transmit the gene to their children, who may have such events. The characteristic sign of the syndrome is a prolonged QT interval on the electrocardiogram (ECG). When the QT is greatly prolonged, the diagnosis is simple. However, in some patients the QT is only borderline prolonged or even normal; in these cases the diagnosis can be difficult. To further complicate early diagnosis, ECGs are not routinely performed in children. Consequently, many patients with this condition go unrecognized until serious symptoms occur. All too often the first event is a cardiac arrest or sudden death.

Research is quite active. Recently, four genes which cause the syndrome have been identified, and others are suspected and being sought. The underlying mechanisms of this disease and the abnormal heart rhythm are being unraveled. The full spectrum of signs and symptoms is being clarified, and it is now evident that there is some diversity in the manifestations of the condition based on the specific gene involved. New treatments are being developed. Physician and public education is increasing. As the remaining genes are identified, genetic analysis will become the most accurate and preferred way to diagnose the condition and additional treatments will be possible. Yet, much remains to be done. Many physicians and most of the public are yet unaware of this silent killer, and misdiagnoses are common.

Often a silver lining exists in clouds of darkness. Thanks to Maryann Anglim and Dr. Walter Allan, such will be the case with Kara's tragedy. Certainly, *Kara Mia* will uplift and strengthen those who must struggle with similar catastrophes. Further, the Long QT syndrome is a very treatable disorder, and the events can be prevented if the disease is recognized early and the proper treatment is instituted. *Kara Mia* will educate and inform and assist in the early and presymptomatic diagnosis and treatment of patients with the Long QT syndrome. Precious lives will be saved as a consequence of this effort.

G. Michael Vincent, M.D.
Chairman, Department of Medicine, LDS Hospital
Professor of Medicine, University of Utah
Salt Lake City, UT

જી જી જી

ა ა ა

Acknowledgments

ა ა ა

The authors would like to acknowledge the help that we received from Anne Lamott's book *bird by bird*. Both of us kept that book near our computers as we wrote and her writing inspired us, got us unstuck, made us laugh, and taught us about life. It had the remarkable effect of eventually making us think we were writers. This particular passage is from the chapter "Someone to Read Your Drafts" and we found it to be particularly true as we solicited editorial assistance from our family and friends.

"...I am suggesting that there may be someone out there in the world...who will read your finished drafts and give you an honest critique, let you know what does and doesn't work, give you some suggestions on things you might take out or things on which you need to elaborate, ways in which to make your piece stronger...I know what a painful feeling it is when you've been working on something forever, and it feels done, and you give your story to someone you hope will validate this and that person tells you it still needs more work. You have to, at this point, question your assessment of this person's character and,...decide whether or not you want them in your life at all. Mostly I think an appropriate first reaction is to think that you don't. But in a while it may strike you as a small miracle that you have someone in your life, whose taste you admire,...who will tell you the truth and help you stay on the straight and narrow, or find your way back to it if you are lost."

So, thank you to Sue Poulin, Marilyn Collins, Lizzie Van Orden, Janet Van Orden, Lynn Baker, Ann Allan, Tom Anglim, Peter Goldfine, Doug Dransfield and Mary Alice Walter.

Your critiques and whole-hearted support encouraged us to continue our writing and not stop until our story was told.

Thanks also to Doug Dransfield for the technological assistance and help with the computerized drawings. You added to the artistic and professional look of the book.

Janice Wright captured the essence of Kara's story in her quilt design on the cover of *Kara Mia*. Thank you very much for all the love and hard work that went into it. We look forward to the day when the quilt design becomes a real quilt.

Thank you to Larry Gorton for the photographic assistance. Also thanks to Diane (Disey) Roussel, R.N. for taking the Christmas photos of Kara on Pediatrics.

Thank you to Joan MacCracken, M.D., author of *The Sun, The Rain and The Insulin*, who willingly shared her experiences and knowledge with us.

Thank you to Medtronic, Inc., not only for having the technologic ability to manufacture implantable cardiac defibrillators, but also for your financial support of our book. Thank you, also, to Jim Winner, our Medtronic representative, for his technical knowledge, for seeing Kara the day of her surgery, and the help with our book.

Thank you to Maine Medical Center for your financial support of *Kara Mia* and for the special brand of care that healed Kara and our family. The people of Maine are fortunate to have your skilled staff available to them.

Thank you to Dr. Michael Vincent for helping a pediatric neurologist and an operating room nurse learn about Long QT syndrome. Thank you for writing the foreword to our book. We join you in your hope of expanding the knowledge of Long QT syndrome.

PART I

SUDDEN LOSS
AND
SLOW RECOVERY

CHAPTER 1

Letters from the Heart
April 10, 1995

৵ ৵ ৵

Dear Kara,

I was very surprised when I heard what had happened to you but I am sure that you will get better. It gets kind of boring around here without cheerful people like you because the kids become quiet. My good friend Michelle, a sixth grader here at Bath Middle School, had to have a heart transplant which I think is much more dangerous than being in a coma. But now she is back healthy and having fun as you will be, too. Everyone misses you and from all I've heard they are taking good care of you. You may not know everyone here as close friends, but I think that what you've been through affected everyone quite a lot. Many students look up to you and can't wait until you come back. At least you don't have to present your science project. Speaking for all of Bath Middle School, hurry and get well because people here will not take "no" for an answer.

Your friend,
Serenity

Hey Kara!

How are you feeling? I hope that you get better real soon. The classes really aren't the same without you. In science there is no one to rub the top of my head. In reading there is no one making that weird noise that you make. And in math, there is no second teacher.

Science really isn't the same without you because you never stop talking. But I don't really mind. It's someone to listen to besides the teacher. And now there is nobody to copy my science answers when you don't have them.

Steph and Heather are taking it really hard. Mrs. Roberts started talking about you and they both started to cry. Even I almost did because you have become a good friend to me this year and no class would be complete without a Kara Anglim in it.

This morning when Mrs. Brunette was reading what the letter from your parents said, she even started crying. So you can see how much everybody misses you. I hope that you get better soon and everybody here loves you.

The person who sits beside you in science,

Tommy

Hey Babe!

You sure know how to scare people. Don't you ever do that again. I miss you so much. I love you a lot. Let's never get in a fight again. Kara, so many people are worried about you and care for you. The whole town of Bath is praying for you. I photocopied *Stairway to Heaven* for you so you can start playing it on the piano when you come home. Chorus is not the same; there is no one here to fool around with. You never know how much you care for a person until something like this happens. I miss you so much. I need you to come back so you can make my mornings at school much brighter. I love you and miss you. Please get better soon and come home. I love you.

Love,

Amy

P. S. You are one of my best friends in the whole wide world.

Kara Bear,

School isn't the same without you. You always brightened my days. Come back soon so you can make me smile and laugh. Everyone cares a lot about you, especially me. You are in my prayers and heart. Everyone is trying to be strong for you, but it is hard to hold back the tears. It makes me glad to know that you are getting better. I was looking at old pictures and saw how many wonderful memories I have of you. Come home soon so we can make more memories and take more pictures. I just want you to know how much I love and care for you and hope you get better soon. I love you.

Kate H.

Kara,

I am so happy to hear that you are getting better everyday. Pretty soon you will be fully recovered. Everyone at school is really concerned. They all miss you. I do, too. It isn't the same here without you. Well, I would have had everyone sign this at school, but I wanted to have one card just from me.

When I found this card it reminded me so much of the day when Kate and I were at your camp in your canoe. We wanted to make it as far across the lake as we could, but we were interrupted from our determination by the water fight that was started.

After thinking about it for awhile, I realized that you have to pull through this one. No matter how big the fight, we always pulled through it together. You are not alone in this battle. I can't speak for everyone else, but I know that I pray every night for you, hoping that you will wake up and be all better. I am sure that I'm not the only one who prays for you. Just remember that even though it sounds really corny, I will always love you! I know that you are strong! You will make it through this.

Love always,
Vanessa

Kara,

I am going to start writing to you in a journal. I think you will want to hear what was going on at the hospital and in life. Friday was a half-day. Remember that deal we had with our parents? That if we went to the dance we would have to stay together on the half-days. Well, my mom made me come home even though you weren't there with me! I went to the dance to TRY and get my mind off you. It didn't work. I was so scared. When I first found out at the track, Angie hugged me and told Amy I was really scary to look at because I was white and shaking and standing there. You really scared me! I guess you really got me back for popping up in your window when you were eating ice cream out of the container. On Sunday we went to church to pray for you—the minister said a special prayer for you. Then I went to visit you! You look so beautiful! You were having a really good face time! Not one single zit and you have a better tan than Guerin or Emily! But it was kind of scary seeing you—you had tubes out of all your fingers, nose, legs and arms. Going there made me realize how much I loved you and missed you. Well, I'll write to you tomorrow.

Love,
Kate B.

Dear Kara,

I don't know you very well, but I've been where you are. I know it's scary and uncomfortable but the feeling you get when you finally come home is wonderful. You notice things you never paid attention to before and normal stuff seems new and exciting. And believe me, I sympathize about the hospital food.

When I was there, the nurses were really caring and considerate. I know that this is really hard for you, but you'll get better soon, so don't worry.

We're signing up for classes today. I can't wait to be a freshman. Open lunch is going to be such a blast! Everyone is worried that all the upperclassmen are going to beat them up. I think that's stupid. The upperclassmen are really nice and I should know because most of my friends are juniors and seniors.

I hope that you get better soon. We really miss you here in Reading. Everybody is concerned for you and we want you to come back soon. Hey, maybe you'll get an extra couple of days vacation. I hope to see you real soon, Kara.

Best wishes,
Lacey

CHAPTER 2

Shocks at the High School Track

తితితి

The time was 3:03 p.m. on April 7, 1995, and Alan Douglass was on duty at the Bath fire station when the call came in that someone had collapsed at the high school track. He and his driver, Robbie Stailing, were off in seconds. It was now 3:04. Alan prides himself on being ALS (Advanced Life Support) trained and certified. He is a full paramedic which means he has the most experience and highest possible ALS rating, and he treats every call as if it needs every bit of that training. The Bath Fire Department ambulance arrived at the track at 3:07 and was waved through the gates by some of the kids. The ambulance lapped the track to the spot where Kara was lying, her coach kneeling beside her and a small knot of kids clustering around her. Alan's first shock was rolling over what he thought was a young boy to see it was a girl. Then a series of other shocks followed. There was the shock of seeing the horrible bluish color of her face, which showed she had not been breathing and was probably in full cardiac arrest. There was the shock of recognizing this girl as Kara Anglim, whom he had known for years. Another shock registered when out of the corner of his eye he caught the expression on the coach's face. The coach had suddenly realized that Kara's life was in danger.

Allowing no time for emotions, Alan acted swiftly. He cleared her airway with his finger, and operating on instinct, he gave her two mouth-to-mouth breaths while Robbie got the Ambu bag out of his pack. Alan then gave Kara a couple of deep chest compressions and put his Lifepac 5 portable monitor/defibrillator on her chest. This device can both read the electrical activity of the heart—the electrocardiogram, or ECG—and deliver a large shock to convert any detected abnormal heart rhythm. Robbie breathed for her with the ventilator bag via a mask. The monitor revealed Kara was in ventricular fibrillation. This rhythm makes the heart behave in a way that produces no coordinated contraction and thus it pumps no blood. It must be converted to normal quickly, otherwise death will soon follow. Alan took a quick tracing for the records and began to charge the defibrillator's capacitor when he realized he did not have a fully charged battery. He had a sinking feeling as he gave Kara a couple more chest compressions and Robbie ventilated her. "Things are not going well," he thought as he changed the battery, "and we need more help." Robbie is an EMT or emergency medical technician. EMTs know basic life support and are trained to assist. Alan realized that they would need more than the two of them if they were going to save Kara.

Alan charged the new battery and delivered the usual 200 joule countershock across Kara's chest. On the monitor her rhythm still showed ventricular fibrillation. She had not converted back to a normal cardiac rhythm. He gave her a couple more chest compressions as he charged the capacitor for another countershock. As he delivered the second shock to Kara, his and her luck changed. Kara came out of ventricular fibrillation and, simultaneously, Mike Drake and David Hudson arrived at the scene. Both were off-duty but had heard the call on their scanners which they keep open for emergencies. Mike has intermediate ALS qualifications. David is a full paramedic. Now David and Alan, the two most experienced men in the town of Bath, were there to help Kara.

Mike laid out the kit Alan would need to place a tube in Kara's trachea to better ventilate her. Robbie took over the chest compressions as Alan moved to Kara's head and smoothly and easily put an endotracheal tube in Kara's trachea. At the same time David slipped a 16-gauge angiocath (a large bore intravenous catheter) in Kara's arm and hooked her up to an intravenous solution of normal saline. Now they had a controlled airway as well as IV access for administering fluids and medications. Alan breathed for Kara through the tube, watching her chest rise with each respiration as he squeezed the Ambu bag. Although she was out of ventricular fibrillation, her heart rhythm between chest compressions was bad. She had a wide, poorly formed ECG, known as an agonal complex, at forty beats per minute, half of the normal rate. This rhythm is only electrical and Kara's heart still was not pumping any blood on its own. David gave her an intravenous injection of epinephrine to try to convert this rhythm to one that would effectively pump blood through Kara's body as Alan and Robbie continued the chest compressions and bag ventilation. Epinephrine, or adrenalin, should have stimulated her heart to return to a normal beat but Kara's rhythm remained agonal. A couple of minutes passed as David prepared a second epinephrine injection and also gave Kara a bolus of atropine, a drug that should speed up the heartbeat.

A second ambulance arrived with more help. Kennie Desmond relieved Robbie on chest compressions and the new members of the team began to prepare the stretcher and ambulance to transport Kara to the hospital emergency room. Her rhythm, between chest compressions still showed the agonal complex at a rate of forty. David gave her a third IV injection of epinephrine. After a minute more of chest compressions and bagging they checked the monitor once more. Kara still maintained an agonal rhythm at forty beats per minute. Alan thought to himself, "I am not sure that we are doing Kara and the Anglims any favors" as they lifted Kara, still lifeless without a real cardiac rhythm and blood pressure, into the ambulance. What he was thinking was that he and David had done thirty full cardiac resuscitations in one year and the six people who survived neurologically intact had all been resuscitated successfully prior to being transported to the hospital. If Kara were to have hope for a meaningful recovery, she needed to respond before transport.

But Alan's final shock came after loading Kara into the ambulance. She suddenly converted to a normal sinus rhythm at one hundred sixty beats per minute. She had a blood pressure and she took a couple of breathes on her own! As the ambulance pulled out of the track, Alan and his team now had some hope that the Anglims' daughter would recover.

9

CHAPTER 3

APRIL 7, 1995

ᘯ ᘯ ᘯ

Our home telephone rang and I ran from the bathroom to answer it in the bedroom. Kara was at track practice, Guerin was in Florida swimming at a national YMCA swim meet and Tom was out shopping for a white shirt to wear to a wedding the next day.

The words were calmly delivered: "Kara passed out on the track." I said back, just as calmly, "I'll be right there." A similar event had occurred to Kara in February and I thought that I knew the drill. I drove hastily to the track which is about three miles from our home expecting to see Kara sitting on the track, surrounded by her ever-attentive friends, waiting for me to take her home.

What I saw was completely different—the ambulance already racing through the track gates and a policeman named Joel telling me not to speed to the hospital. "Don't worry, I won't," I assured him. I was thinking that when I arrived at the emergency room, Kara would be resting on a stretcher sipping a Coke, eating a popsicle, surrounded now by a bevy of nurses attending to her every whim.

But when I arrived at the emergency room door, I could sense that the ambulance had been parked quickly and that Kara had been just as quickly rushed into the emergency room. I haphazardly parked my car off to the side of the hospital entrance as fear and worry were replacing my vision of Kara sipping a Coke. I ran into the emergency room and pulled back the dividing curtain to see Kara lying on a stretcher in what I knew in my heart was critical condition.

She was, indeed, surrounded by a bevy of nurses and technicians but she was intubated and a respiratory therapist was breathing for her. She was attached to a cardiac monitor, an automatic blood pressure cuff, an oximeter, had two IVs running, one in each arm, and a catheter in her bladder. Being a nurse, I knew the questions to ask. "Did you defibrillate her?" "Yes, two times," came the answer. "She was in v-fib when we arrived," said the EMTs, "and then she went into an agonal rhythm. We didn't think that we would get her back."

Now my observations were a mixture of mother and nurse as she lay so dependent upon the skill of others in the emergency room. She had on her red and white Umbro shorts. I remembered the day I bought them. Someone's brown plaid flannel shirt lay beneath her. I wondered whose shirt it was. Her rings were still on her fingers. I thought I had better take them off in case her fingers got swollen. Her chest had slight red marks on it from the defibrillator. "How can this be happening?" I asked myself. She was so dirty from the track. I kept trying to wipe the dirt off as I talked to her and told her that I loved her, as I begged her not to leave me. I watched the monitor and listened to the interplay among the emergency room team members.

Then came the questions. "Where is your husband?" "Out buying a shirt." "Where?" "I don't know." I felt as if I were a bad wife because I didn't know where my husband was. I wondered if they knew where their husbands were all of the time. "Do you want the priest to come?" "Yes." By asking this question, I knew that the emergency room staff thought that Kara might die. "Can we call someone to be with you?" "Yes, get Linda."

There I sat on a stool as I watched these people try to save my daughter's life. I saw the dopamine drip, heard the blood gas results, saw the chest X-ray and pieced together what was happening before my eyes. I knew exactly what Kara was facing and that her future lay somewhere between death and a complete recovery and that there was a long continuum between those two points where she might come to rest.

Suddenly Linda Coes appeared and her arms were around me. Linda is my best friend and we have worked together for years in the operating room. I observed the look of

11

shock and amazement on her face as she absorbed the scenario before us. Linda always knows what to do and she mobilized herself to sit by Kara's head and whisper into her ear. I didn't need to hear the words because I knew that she telling Kara not to be afraid and that she was going to be fine. At one point, Linda looked at me and said, "What happened?" I couldn't answer her because I had no explanation. I just looked at her and said quietly so no one else could hear, "She is going to die." But Linda wouldn't allow that thought. "We are not going to let her," she said.

Next the lanky, craggy Catholic priest appeared in the emergency room. He looked like Ichabod Crane. It was amazing to me that he was there to give the Last Rites to my daughter. I remembered learning the seven sacraments in second grade. Then Last Rites were called Extreme Unction, and I remember not paying too much attention to this particular sacrament because, after all, it was the last sacrament we learned and it seemed reserved for old people. The priest prayed over Kara, his voice more distinctive than the hum of the working voices. I heard him say, "Forgive Kara her sins," and I remember saying, "She didn't even have a chance to make a sin." I immediately felt apologetic for being cynical. Even at that early stage I knew that cynicism wasn't an emotion that would help our family through this. The priest mumbled some words of encouragement to me and wafted off just as a benevolent spirit should.

The cast of main characters remained fairly constant in the emergency room but new ones kept entering, exiting and then reappearing. Dr. Rebecca Chagrasulis was the emergency room team leader and I knew that Kara was in capable hands with her. She had taught the Advanced Cardiac Life Support course many times and I had great respect for her skill. Dr. David Enright, Kara's pediatrician, now appeared at her feet. I was glad to see him. He is a serious and hard-thinking doctor and his presence could only help. I didn't even greet him. My first words to him were, "Could you call Dr. Allan?" Dr. Walter Allan is a pediatric neurologist at Maine Medical Center, and he had been Kara's doctor for five years. I knew that we were going to need his help to assess Kara's neurologic status, and I just hoped that he was available.

Laboratory technicians, X-ray technicians, respiratory therapists, nurses, doctors and EMTs all played their parts. They were in and out, on the telephone, and arguing politely with each other. I was wondering if Kara were having a "near death experience" which I had heard people who had survived catastrophic events describe. Was she floating above us looking down and observing? I looked up but all that I saw was the ceiling. "Don't be weird," I told myself.

Kara's condition was extremely critical but she was stable enough for the team to consider transferring her to Maine Medical Center which is thirty-five miles away in Portland. I knew that they were trying to decide how to get her there in the safest and most efficient way possible and there was definite controversy over this issue. All that I really cared about was that I would be allowed to ride with her in the ambulance and hold her. I wasn't sure how much longer I would be able to have her and I wanted to spend every moment with her.

The decision took a while to make, but once it was made, Kara was quickly transferred into the ambulance, and she and I and Dr. Enright, an emergency room nurse and two EMTs climbed into the back of the ambulance. Linda knew the EMTs and they allowed her to ride up in the front with the drivers. I was so grateful that Linda was there. I knew that she would be able to be strong in case I couldn't be. Kara felt so cold and before we drove off I asked the nurse for some blankets. A mother's job is to keep her children warm.

As we were leaving, a nurse told me that they had located Tom at home and that he would meet us in Portland at the hospital. He was just starting to cook a Chinese stir-fry dish that Kara had requested for dinner. I felt that bad feeling in my stomach in sympathy for Tom. At least I was with Kara and knew what was going on with her. I was part of the process and the hope. All Tom had was his imagination and his fears. Maybe he did not have any hope. "Dear God, help us be strong," I prayed, "and help him not be too scared."

CHAPTER 4

With Grace and Maturity

୬ ୬ ୬

The ride to Portland was quick and I only remember asking three things. First I asked Dr. Enright what the date was. He looked at his watch and replied, "April 7th." I knew that date would now be as memorable as a birthday or an anniversary. The second thing I asked was "Do you think that Kara is getting too much fluid?" as I observed frothy secretions project from her endotracheal tube. I didn't listen to the answer as I started to imagine how hard it must be to balance enough fluids to sustain a blood pressure but not produce pulmonary edema. I couldn't watch how fast the IVs were dripping because the motion of the ambulance made it impossible. The third question was "Where are we?" "At Dexter Shoe," came the answer. That meant we were in Brunswick with another half-hour until we arrived at Maine Medical Center. Mostly I kept holding Kara. Her arms kept wanting to hang over the edges of the stretcher and I knelt by her side keeping her arms safely tucked in close to her body.

Sometimes I watched the cars on the highway. In second grade at Catholic school we learned to say a prayer whenever we heard a siren or saw an ambulance or fire truck. Someone was in distress and needed our sweet and innocent prayers. I still whisper a prayer although my prayers now are not nearly so sweet nor so innocent. For all those people in cars driving with us on the highway, April 7 was an ordinary day. I'm sure none of them imagined that inside was a fourteen-year-old girl who only hours before had been a silly and carefree eighth grader. Maybe they knew from their second grade teachers that they were supposed to pray for us.

We arrived at the hospital and parked at the emergency room entrance which resembled a big concrete loading dock. As I hopped out of the ambulance, I saw Tom standing outside. He looked calm. That is a good trait, to be calm in the presence of an emergency. By this time he knew that Kara had collapsed at track practice and that she had survived a cardiac arrest, but those were the only two details of which he was aware. I didn't know much more than that. With his arm around me, we watched, silent and resigned, as the EMTs lifted Kara from the ambulance.

Dr. Sandy Bagwell, who was to be Kara's physician in the Special Care Unit, met the ambulance, and I could see her quietly assessing Kara and scanning the situation. There were probably other people there but I only remember Tom and Dr. Bagwell. We went through some doors and into a big steel elevator. Once the doors opened on the upper floor, we traveled down a long hallway, into the Special Care Unit, and then into the room assigned to Kara. A male voice asked me, "Does she have asthma?" As I answered, "No," I thought gratefully that at least there was one problem that she didn't have. Dr. Bagwell asked me, "Does she have any siblings?" "Yes," I said, "a sister." "Where is she?" "In Florida at a swim meet." "When will she be home?" "On Sunday." At the time I couldn't understand why she was so interested in Guerin when Kara was the critically ill sister. It took me many days to realize that it was because Kara's condition was so precarious that our whole family should be together while we could. In case...just in case.

The drapes of the cubicle were shut and the door was closed and I knew the flurry of activity that was going on in there. I didn't mind not being in the room. Right now Kara needed their medical expertise more than she needed my mothering expertise. I think that I work better as a nurse when I don't have family members observing my technical skills and probably the Special Care Unit staff felt the same way.

As we waited, our friend Sandy Zimmerman appeared. He is a Special Care Unit physician and we know him from various activities at the Bath YMCA. He was the first person who made me smile since the phone call came. Linda was telling him that she had been at the beauty shop getting her hair streaked when someone tracked her down and told her that I needed her. He glanced at her half done hair-do and said, "I hope that you didn't have to pay." Both Linda and I looked a fright.

Next a little dark-haired social worker suddenly stood in front of me. She had on big thick-framed black glasses. They resembled the glasses that Aristotle Onassis wore. I had to concentrate hard on what she was saying because I kept looking at those glasses. She told me a number of things but I didn't absorb most of them. I pretended that I did and kept saying "Yes, okay" to everything. The only things I did remember was that we could stay overnight in a Portland hotel for a cheaper rate if we chose and that we could get some temporary cash if we needed money. I sensed that we were part of a system that was set in motion at the medical center whenever a catastrophic illness occurred.

Then came a phone call for me at the nurses' station. "Hello," I said tentatively because I had no idea who could possibly be calling me. It was a church lady telling me that the Catholic church in Bath had started a prayer chain for Kara. I wondered what a prayer chain was, but I knew it was something for which I should be grateful. Maybe they planned to pray all night for Kara—they would be exhausted by the morning.

Dr. Allan appeared. Over the years that he had been Kara's doctor, I had developed some sense of his personality and a definite sense of his skill. I was so glad to see him and so relieved that he was available to help Kara that I gave him a hug. There is no delicate way to say it—we needed him to tell us if there were any hope for neurologic recovery for Kara. I asked him, "Will you help us make the right decisions?" He said he would and he did. Then he went into the room to examine Kara and told us that he would talk to us afterwards.

Dr. Maribeth Hourihan was already in Kara's room. She is a pediatric cardiologist. She is blond, cute and smart and I knew that Kara would love having her as her doctor. She introduced herself to us and told us her plan which was to do an echocardiogram and see how Kara's heart looked after the insult that it had suffered. She was also looking for reasons for the cardiac arrest. She, too, told us that she would talk to us after the echocardiogram.

I knew that Kara was getting excellent care, and now all we could do was wait for the experts to give their opinions and plans. Tom, Linda and I went into the hallway outside the unit to give the doctors and nurses the time they needed and maybe allow ourselves the time to take a deep breath. That was not to be, however, because a crowd of friends awaited us, wanting news of Kara's condition and hoping to help.

Rufus Coes, Linda's husband, said to us, "What are you going to do about Guerin?" I was thinking that we should just let her enjoy her last day in Florida, let her drive home with the rest of her swim teammates and then help her deal with the reality of Kara's sudden illness on Sunday. Luckily Rufus was being more realistic and analytical than either Tom or I and he said, "You have to tell her the news before she hears it from anyone else. Also, we have to make plane reservations for her so that she can fly home as soon as possible." He said it so authoritatively and so assuredly that I knew that he must be right. He dialed the phone number as I pondered the correct manner and the right words to tell Guerin the devastating news. This is not something that is covered in Dr. Spock. But I did know that my attitude would become her attitude and I had to be honest but allow her the luxury of optimism and hope. First Linda spoke to Guerin as I tried to collect my words and thoughts and then Linda passed the phone to me. Guerin probably knew immediately the depth of the tragedy our family was facing because my voice was so strange. I sounded strange even to myself.

Guerin was eighteen, a senior in high school, and her life was a frenzy of college plans, swimming, friends and fun. Now she would have to become an adult instantly. I told her the story and she handled it well until I told her that Kara was presently in a coma. She started crying and asked me if Kara was going to die. I told her that Kara was critically ill and that everyone was working hard to keep her alive but that no one knew the answer to that question right now. Then her crying turned into uncontrollable sobs. I told her that Tom and I were holding ourselves together and that she had to do the same. Sadness and fear were emotions that we couldn't deny but we all had to handle them with grace and maturity. I expected that of her and in the weeks to come she did not disappoint me. Plans were made for her to fly home to Maine the next day and soon she would play a big part in Kara's recovery.

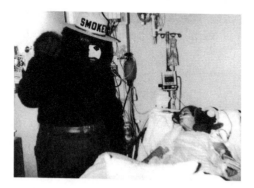

Kara in coma during Smokey the Bear's rounds in the Special Care Unit.

CHAPTER 5

A Doctor's Impressions
by Walter Allan, M.D.

৬৯ ৬৯ ৬৯

It was a Friday afternoon and I was seeing the last of my patients when Mary-Lou, my secretary, put through the call from Dave Enright. "Walter, I am in the emergency room with Kara Anglim," he said in a calm voice. "She was at track practice and had what was described as a seizure. By the time the EMTs arrived she was in v-fib and had to be countershocked twice..."

While he was in midsentence, I knew this was not a call about a simple seizure. When he mentioned that Kara had been at track practice, I felt something much worse had happened. My most vivid memory of the conversation is that I was a step ahead of what Dave was saying. I was thinking about Kara's last visit with me in March. I had uncertainty about the cause of her spells. This thought and its implications were slowly making their way forward from the back of my mind as Dave was telling me the details.

"Shit, Dave, this was an arrest. It wasn't a seizure. This doesn't happen after a seizure. I have always thought that things weren't clear cut here. Jesus Christ!"

"I think you're right. She's in sinus rhythm now and her vital signs are okay but she's posturing and tremulous. Do you think these movements might be seizures?" he asked. Kara's diagnosis had been epilepsy and he must have been wondering how I could be so sure Kara had a completely different medical problem.

"She has extensor posturing from anoxic injury because of the arrest. It's not a seizure. You don't get v-fib from a seizure," I said, sure of my thoughts about what must have happened. I was still stuck on the idea that Kara had nearly died from a cardiac arrest. I had no idea why Kara would have had a cardiac arrest but there were more pressing issues to discuss. "Are her pupils working?"

He answered, "Yes," and we proceeded to make arrangements for Kara to come down to Maine Medical Center. I had to make some calls to the Special Care Unit and Sandy Bagwell, the chief of Pediatric Critical Care Medicine, to get things arranged, and I told him that I would call him back. Then he added, "Maryann is here and wants to be sure you will be there to assess Kara." I said, "Of course, I'll be there."

I called Sandy and said, "Sandy, Dave Enright has a patient of mine in the Bath ER with a v-fib arrest. She has reactive pupils and is in sinus rhythm. They want to transfer her down. I think the best thing is to let them transfer her rather than wait for our team to go to get her, but you should call him." Then I said what I have told a hundred-plus colleagues, residents, nurses, therapists, administrators, typists, cleaning ladies and passersby when I first relate Kara's story: "Kara is fourteen and one of my favorite patients. I've known her since she was eight and her mother would send me a Christmas card with her photo each year. It would say things such as: 'To our favorite doctor'."

I explained to Sandy that I had followed Kara for epilepsy, but when I last saw her in my office I was wondering if that was really the diagnosis. Now we knew it was cardiac. She said she would get the pediatric cardiologists involved and asked what I thought the outlook was.

"There is no telling. I've got to see her first and get an EEG. Dave says she's stable but he wants to get her down here as soon as possible since we don't really know what happened." I ended the conversation saying, "This is going to be tough," thinking about Kara and Maryann and those Christmas cards. "I'll meet you in SCU if you page me when they get here."

I finished the phone call and went out to get my last patient. I stopped by Mary-Lou's desk and said, "Dave Enright says Kara Anglim had a cardiac arrest and is comatose up in the Bath ER." She looked struck by the news. Mary-Lou also

20

especially liked Kara and Maryann. I finished in the office and then went to the Neonatal Intensive Care Unit to look at cranial ultrasound scans and see if there were any neurologic problems they needed me to assess. I began telling Kara's story to Doug Dransfield, my closest friend and head of neonatology. I think I tell these stories to help sort them out in my own mind. I was thinking of what I would see and say in the next hours when I got beeped. It was Sandy Bagwell. Kara had arrived at the Special Care Unit.

I remember coming into the unit and seeing Kara's parents. Maryann gave me a hug and said how relieved she was that I was there. I met Tom for the first time and shook his hand. I asked them both to go out of the room so that I could examine Kara and then we would talk about her condition. Maribeth Hourihan, one of our pediatric cardiologists, was already there examining Kara.

On my exam Kara had intact brain stem reflexes and reactive pupils—both good signs. She had nearly constant tremor of all muscle groups, as Dave had described. These were the movements he thought might be seizures. However, when you pinched her, she had slight flexion of her arms. It wasn't good, but it wasn't hopeless. I vaguely remember Dave being there and speaking to him but mostly I was trying to think of how to talk about all of this with Maryann and Tom.

I met with the Anglims in the room we use for teaching purposes, just around the corner from Kara's room. I started by asking Maryann what had happened at the track and in the emergency room. After listening to be sure I had the full story, I tried to give the Anglims my best idea of how things were at the moment.

"What matters most, immediately after an arrest, is whether the person regains pupillary response," I said. "Dave told me that Kara had reactive pupils in the ER, which is a good sign. When I looked at her just now, she had intact corneal reflexes and a gag reflex as well. When you pinch her, she flexes her arms slightly which is also a good sign. But, of course, she is in a coma, which is never good. There is statistically-based information about the outlook from the six-hour post arrest exam. So we'll look at all this again in a few hours. Meanwhile, we'll get an EEG—an electroencephalogram or brain wave test—to be sure that those tremors aren't seizures. I don't think that they are but we need to look with an EEG. Right now, I think we should be cautiously optimistic since she has a better exam at three hours than she had in the Bath ER. We'll know better at six hours."

Maribeth had come with me to talk with the Anglims about Kara's heart and her sudden cardiac arrest. She said she was not sure what had caused the arrest and that there were more tests to be done. But, she said that Kara's heart did not look damaged and was pumping well at present.

At six hours, the EEG showed no sign of seizures but there was generalized slowing. That couldn't tell us much either way, but she did have brain waves. Her exam showed better flexor movements in the arms and the nurses noted spontaneous eye opening. All of this was encouraging, and speaking statistically, I thought that Kara had at least a fifty percent chance of making a recovery to a good level. By a good level of recovery I meant being able to return to school, perhaps with help, but maybe even recovering completely. I did my best to give the Anglims some hope.

CHAPTER 6

A Mother's Impressions

ଏକ ଏକ ଏକ

Tom and I and our ever-growing entourage waited in the hallway near the pay telephone for the doctors to complete their examinations of Kara. We made quite a few phone calls across the country to family members to inform them of Kara's collapse, and I learned how hard it is to use an AT&T calling card when one is upset. Someone should tell them that it is just too complicated to dial all of those numbers in a crisis. AT&T should develop an easier system made especially for bereft people.

It seems that we waited for about an hour, and I felt ambivalent about talking to the doctors and hearing their assessments, opinions and plans. I dreaded hearing anything negative and hopeless, but I knew that perhaps what I would hear would be positive and hopeful. It didn't matter how I felt because we would have to deal with the reality of Kara's condition whether the news was good or bad. Suddenly Tom and I were in a freezing and empty classroom with Dr. Allan and Dr. Hourihan. I was so cold and so scared and so nervous. I was holding Tom's hand tightly, and I must have been breaking his fingers or at least causing some nerve damage, but he was probably too numb to notice.

It must have been difficult for Dr. Allan and Dr. Hourihan to talk to us. We are parents who tried hard to do everything correctly as we raised our daughters. There was always a part of me which thought that if I loved them, fed them correctly, kept them safe, gave them everything they needed but didn't spoil them, encouraged good morals, read to them, kept them clean and warm, helped their educational and cultural development and taught them how to laugh and see the humor in life that we would be immune to such a disaster. We probably were not that different from the types of parents that those two doctors are. Now we were experiencing every parent's nightmare. I imagine that we were a fairly heartbreaking image. But doctors have to separate the emotional from the physical, and they were able to give us the facts of Kara's condition and allow us the hope of a recovery for her. That was the most important message I received from the meeting in that cold empty room. There was hope and maybe my heart didn't need to feel as cold and empty as that room.

First Dr. Allan spoke about Kara's neurologic status and its implication for her recovery. Neurology, to me, is a complex, confusing maze of basal ganglia and neurons, but he spoke simply and clearly of pupillary reaction, corneal and gag reflexes, flexor movement and response to pain and how all these were allowing us cautious optimism with the emphasis on the word "cautious." The scheduled EEG would answer our most fearful question: "Would Kara have brain waves?"

Then Dr. Hourihan gave us her assessment of Kara's cardiac arrest. She said simply, "Your daughter experienced what we call sudden death." I remember gasping audibly and saying, "Dear God!" I know that I was biting my lip so I wouldn't cry. I knew about sudden death from the Advanced Cardiac Life Support course that I am required to take every other year, but in my naiveté, I had considered it a problem of unfortunate older individuals, not my daughter. Sudden death is a medical term that encompasses a number of different diagnoses, and in Kara's case Dr. Hourihan felt the cause was an electrical disorder of the heart muscle, possibly one called Long QT syndrome. She had already done the echocardiogram of Kara's heart and told us that it was mildly abnormal which she expected, and she would repeat it tomorrow at which time she expected it to have returned to normal. Then she spoke about treatment. Drug therapy, pacemaker and implanted defibrillator were all mentioned. She concluded, "We will protect her heart so that this will never happen again." That statement was aimed at Kara's future so it seemed a positive way to end this meeting.

24

We went back into the unit to see Kara again. The nurses had her all cleaned up and her hair combed but there was no denying the fact that this was a sick child. Now, in addition to all the equipment that monitored her in the emergency room at Bath, there was also an arterial line in her left wrist, a triple lumen catheter in her right groin, a nasogastric tube, a ventilator and a temperature probe. Linda and I examined the insertion sites of every invasive monitor and tube. In the operating room, we are used to our patients being heavily monitored and sometimes you cannot separate the nurse from the mother. We checked all of the numbers and tracings on the monitor. We might not know neurology or cardiology, but we do know monitors. Despite the fact that Kara was surrounded by all of the accouterments of a severe illness, she looked just as pretty as Sleeping Beauty lying in the bed. Her face was serene and peaceful and her body relaxed. If only the fairy tale could come true and a princely kiss could wake her and make her well.

Slowly, all of our friends went home and just Tom and I were left with Kara. I did not want to leave her side, even though I knew the doctors and nurses were taking good care of her, but I knew from my own nursing experience, that the parents of sick children need their rest, too. By the time we both got into the car to drive back to an empty house, we did know that the EEG showed Kara had brain waves and, for us, it meant we would press forward with all our strength and heart to help her recover. The night seemed endless. I did not sleep at all that night. As I listened to Tom snore, I couldn't understand how he could sleep. When I asked him the next morning how he could fall asleep so easily, he simply told me, "I was tired." I had better read that book *Men are from Mars, Women are from Venus* by John Gray, Ph.D. because it must be true.

CHAPTER 7
Like Patterns for a Quilt

అ అ అ

Eventually Saturday morning did arrive and as I rode in the car down to Portland, I wrote a letter to the Bath Middle School staff and students. All of Kara's friends and teammates had witnessed her collapse and subsequent resuscitation, and I could only imagine what a dramatic impression this had left on their fragile adolescent psyches. I felt a responsibility to help them through this tumultuous experience by sharing the medical facts of Kara's condition, offering them hope for her recovery and encouraging them to be courageous and adopt brave attitudes. This set the pattern for my weekly letters to the school community, and everyone became outraged if I missed a week of newsy medical updates. It became only one of many patterns in the quilt of Kara's recovery.

A second pattern was the linoleum floor at Maine Medical Center. As I walked through the corridor from the front entrance, past the portrait of L.L. Bean and up to the Special Care Unit, I eventually came to a ramp with nonskid black adhesive tapes arranged in a symmetrical formation. That was my signal that the unit was just around the corner, that Kara really was critically ill and that I really was living a nightmare. My stomach would start to hurt. That happened every day for the nine days that Kara was in the Special Care Unit. I think that if I should go and look at that floor pattern again it would provoke the same stomachache.

The Special Care Unit at Maine Medical Center was true to its name. Not only did the unit give Kara the special critical care that she needed, but it also gave Tom and me the special emotional care that we required through this time. Linda was with us for much of it and together she and I timidly asked the nurses if they would let us give Kara her first bath. I knew that I would feel better if I could just do this one task, but I knew that I needed Linda to help me through it. Kara was still in a coma with a ventilator breathing for her, and she still had multiple tubes, IVs and catheters. The nurses didn't really know us, but I think that they used that sixth sense all the best nurses seem to have and allowed us to be the mothers we are. They were still definitely in charge. They checked the water temperature and watched how we turned and positioned Kara as we washed off all of the track dirt left over from the day before, but they trusted us and let us do it.

Operating room nurses are not bed bath specialists. Actually, I only remember giving one complete bath to a patient in all of the twenty-three years that I have worked in the operating room. Probably we were very slow and clumsy, but Kara was clean. Then the nurses gave us the ultimate compliment, that we were so capable that we could wash Kara's hair the next day. Linda and I looked at each other with terror in our eyes because we couldn't even begin to imagine the complexities of such a task. Certainly assisting with open heart surgery would be easier than giving a shampoo to a comatose patient! But the next day we learned one more new skill and gave Kara her first shampoo, even though it took as much planning as it probably takes to launch a space shuttle. One of the few things I could do for her then was to brush her hair and try to get the paste from her many EEGs out of it. Kara has beautiful thick brown hair with blonde streaks in it, and I spent hours in the unit just brushing her hair. Whenever I didn't know what else to do, I brushed her hair. I hope that it felt good to her because it felt good to me. The important pattern here is that, despite how sick Kara was, I was being allowed to be her mom and take care of her.

Of course, there were the patterns of the doctors' visits. Every morning Dr. Allan would examine Kara before his office hours and again every evening. Each morning he would greet us and get our impressions of Kara's condition and then ask us to leave her room so he could determine her neurologic status. I would gladly leave because I knew he was asking her to do such simple things: open her eyes, sit up, hold her head upright, look at him.

In those early days of her illness, it was hard for me to see what she could do. It was easier for me to see what she couldn't do and that was painful and sad. As I got to know Dr. Allan better, he would tell me that I didn't need to leave the room while he examined her but I always did. It was cowardly of me, I know, but I think that it saved me an ocean of tears. With his experience, he could see things that I couldn't and it was my choice for him to tell me about them rather than for me to try to observe them myself. He always had the correct blend of optimism and realism and he gave me the courage to trust that Kara would achieve some reasonable level of neurological recovery.

There were so many doctors involved in Kara's complicated medical care. Dr. Bagwell is the physician in charge of the pediatric patients in the Special Care Unit. It was her job to insure that Kara remained medically stable as she monitored her heart rate and ECG, blood pressure, kidney function, fluid intake, respirations, central venous pressure, oxygen saturation, temperature and overall welfare. With Kara, this was a full-time job. Dr. Bagwell was smart, clear-thinking and professional in her manner and attitudes, and I learned a lot from observing her. At one point, Kara's arterial line had stopped working, and the question became whether to replace it or totally discontinue it. Dr. Bagwell thought aloud as she balanced the good versus the bad of keeping in an invasive monitoring device and decided that at this point in Kara's recovery the bad outweighed the good and discontinued the arterial line altogether. It seemed a simple and effective technique for dealing with medical decisions as well as general life decisions. "I'll have to remember this style and try to be more like her," I thought to myself. Dr. Bagwell also always held out hope for me to trust that a good recovery for Kara was possible. She told me about a patient of hers who had a brain injury as severe as Kara's and with many of the same problems who returned to the hospital to visit Dr. Bagwell, showing a report card filled with fine grades. I looked forward to the day when we could do that, too.

The cardiac doctors were hard at work consulting with each other and their colleagues in other cities about a diagnosis and treatment plan for Kara. Her cardiac problems just would not easily fall into any one category, and they, too, were weighing the positives and negatives of different therapies. Kara's echocardiogram was back to normal by Saturday, but that didn't help solve the problem of future protection for Kara's heart. Tom and I met Dr. Joel Cutler whose specialty is the electrophysiology of the heart. Dr. Cutler is tall, thin and serious, and he went to Hampshire College, an innovative New England college, so we knew that there must be a creative and inventive bent to his mind. He spoke about Kara's arrhythmia and the fact that while he was suspecting the problem was Long QT syndrome, didactic proof didn't exist yet. Kara was still critically ill and while it was premature to actually do any invasive treatments or testing, it was time to be thinking and planning what the next steps in Kara's health plan would be. He spoke of pacemakers, implantable defibrillators and drug therapy and said that her future might hold any or all of these therapies. He also spoke of electrophysiologic studies and heart muscle biopsies, and I was glad that we had yet another smart and skilled person to help Kara find her way back to good health.

Kara also had a physiatrist, which is the '90s term for a rehabilitation physician, in addition to physical therapists, respiratory therapists, occupational therapists, a speech therapist, a social worker, a psychiatric nurse, a recreational therapist and a neuropsychologist.

More than any help that I could have gotten from a psychiatrist or psychologist was the support I received from the Special Care Unit nurses. They have dealt with so many families in tragic situations that they know the right words to say and the right things to do. I think that they observed us through the glass walls of Kara's room more than I realized; they didn't only watch Kara, they watched Tom and Guerin and me. One day Kara and I were alone in her room. I had my back to the window and was sitting in a chair leaning on the side rail of her bed. Suddenly the entire scenario seemed so unbelievable, but so real and sad, that I just closed my eyes, put my head on the side rail and cried. I thought that I was being discrete but I couldn't fool those nurses. Quickly Kara's primary nurse was there with her arm around me. I told her that I had cried so many tears that my contact lenses were all foggy and that I had to stop crying so I could see again. "Or you could just wear your glasses and cry all that you want," she said. And then there was the time that Kara was dressed in a yellow hospital gown. Guerin commented casually that yellow was not a color that looked good on Kara and the next time I saw Kara she had on a blue hospital gown. These nurses were highly skilled and busy individuals, yet they took the time to listen to a teenager's comment about her sister and let her have one small element of control in her sister's care. I don't think that a psychiatrist could have done a better job.

All of these people with all of their different skills and personalities made up the complicated and colorful patterns which comprised the quilt of Kara's first stages of recovery.

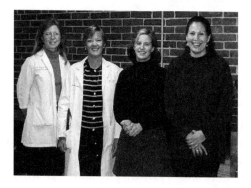

Three blondes and a brunette: Dr. Bagwell, Dr. Hourihan and Dr. DeCorey-Woronoff with Kara at Christmas 1996.

CHAPTER 8

A Sister's Impressions
by Guerin Elizabeth Anglim

✎ ✎ ✎

"Eleventh place goes to Long Reach Swim Club of Bath, Maine..." the announcer's voice was drowned out by our excited screams.

"Oh my God! I can't even believe that we did it," I said as my eyes filled with tears of happiness. Eleanor, Eliza, Katrine and I all hugged as the shock that our 200-free relay team had made it to finals settled in our minds. What that meant was that we were going to swim that night again with the fastest relay teams in the nation. It was the first relay from Maine to ever have made it to the finals at Nationals and it was something that we had been working toward all season. Our coaches, Jay and Todd, were very proud of us and the rest of our team was also.

Our relay team was on cloud nine for the rest of the beautiful, sunny, Florida day. We all went out to lunch at Joe Belair's, our favorite spot, and then Eleanor, Eliza and I relaxed in the hotel. Katrine was only thirteen years old and had tons of energy so she played in the ocean all that afternoon.

Before we knew it, it was time to go back to the Ft. Lauderdale Hall of Fame Pool to swim. We all had on our matching black paper suits and blue caps. We dove in to warm up and it was exciting just to be warming up with all the other swimmers who had made it to finals. The 200-free relay was the first event so we didn't have much time to be nervous. Our coach, Jay, gave us a pep talk and then we gathered behind our starting block to wait. It was getting pretty cold because the sun was going down and we stretched to try and stay warm. We didn't talk much because the butterflies had begun. We just gave each other a few wishes of good luck and warnings not to false start.

A whistle blew and before I knew it, Eleanor was climbing onto the block. "Take your mark...BEEP!!!" And Eleanor was off. Then Katrine swam her leg of the relay and next Eliza dove into the water. I was last and as I stood on the block my body felt as if it were floating and I never wanted to leave the block. But Eliza touched the wall and I had to go. I dove in and swam as fast as I possibly could until I finished. I looked up at the scoreboard and saw that we had come in sixteenth. I hauled myself out of the water and we all congratulated each other because coming in sixteenth meant that we had won points for our team. We walked back to our team and everyone hugged us as we got more congratulations. Jay showed us our splits and then told us to get ready for the award ceremony. We went into the locker room and changed out of our uncomfortable wet suits and felt relief that the four-day meet was over.

Walking onto the award stand was so fun. It was a dream come true and the ribbon that each of us received was humungous.

Once our entire team had piled into our red van we decided to celebrate by going out to dinner at the Olive Garden. Katrine needed to go back to the hotel to get her money so we made a quick stop. We were all waiting in the van and Jay came out and told me that I had a phone call. I was excited to get a call and joked that maybe it was the hot guy that had won all the events at Nationals whom we had drooled over the whole meet.

"Hello," I said into the receiver.

"Hi Guerin. It's your Aunt Linda. How are you?"

"Oh, I'm great. We just got back from finals and we got sixteenth. You should see how big the ribbons are." I thought that it was a little weird that Aunt Linda was calling me but not that weird because her daughter, Emily, was also in Florida with me.

"Well, I have some bad news for you. It's about Kara. Here's your mom."

"Hi Guerin." My mom's voice sounded strained and worried.

"Is Kara OK? Did she have a seizure again?"

"Yes, but this was a really bad seizure where she stopped breathing and now she's in a coma."

"Oh my God! Is she going to wake up?" As soon as I heard the word coma I started crying. Jay ran over to me and hugged me. The rest of the conversation is a blur. I remember Mom telling me that Kara might die and that I was going to fly home the next morning with Emily. Then I gave the phone to Jay so that he could make the arrangements for me to fly home because I was too upset to remember any details. I went out to the van to get Emily to tell her what happened because she is like a sister to me. Emily quietly began crying.

Emily and I decided to go out to eat with the rest of the team because the thought of sitting alone in the hotel was depressing. Once again we were all in the van, but this time it was silent except for my sniffles. We arrived at the restaurant and that brought another wave of tears because the last time Emily and I had been at the Olive Garden we had been with Kara on her fourteenth birthday. Aunt Linda had told the waiter that it was Kara's birthday and he brought out a little cake while all the wait staff sang to her. Kara loved it as soon as she got over the surprise. And now Kara was in the hospital—it seemed so unreal. I just wanted to see her so that I could tell her I loved her and to get better.

It was really hard to fall asleep that night. As I lay in bed I wondered why this had happened because it didn't make any sense. Kara had seizures before and this never happened. Then, I got paranoid that my heart was going to suddenly stop. Finally, I fell asleep knowing that my life was never going to be the same.

When the wake-up call rang early the next morning it took me a minute to remember that Kara was in the hospital. Coincidentally, Emily and I were on the same flight as Katrine Alcaide and her dad. The rest of the team was driving back in the van later on that day. I did some last minute packing and took a quick shower. Soon Mr. Alcaide was knocking on the door. I said good-bye to everyone and then we hopped into his rental car.

It turned out to be the longest plane ride of my life

even though Mr. Alcaide had gotten us into first class. I tried to sleep because I felt exhausted but I could only doze for short intervals. I kept picturing Kara in the hospital and wondering if she was going to recover. I knew that she wasn't going to die because she was so tough and strong. I was just worried about the brain damage. I tried not to think about Kara but it was impossible. I didn't want Emily and Katrine to know that I was crying so I pretended I was sleeping and covered my face with my jacket.

We finally landed in Portland, Maine, where Uncle Rufus, Julia (Emily's twin sister), and Sam (Julia's boyfriend) were waiting for us. I looked at everyone's sad red eyes and began crying again. Julia hugged me and mothered me even though she is two years younger than I am and physically much smaller. Emily and I said good-bye to the Alcaides and Uncle Rufus drove us to Maine Medical Center. My dad was waiting for me outside and my Grampy was there, too. I was cold in my cutoffs and tee shirt. We walked into the hospital and my dad told me that I should say "hi" to my grandfather since I hadn't seen him since Christmas. I did even though I didn't feel as if I wanted to speak to anyone. That was the first time that I saw him crying. It seemed as if we walked forever and all of a sudden my mom was there hugging me. She walked me the rest of the way to Kara's room and told me what to expect so I wouldn't be too surprised. She told me not to let Kara hear me cry and just to talk to her as if she were awake.

When I saw Kara, I couldn't believe my eyes. There was my sister lying in that bed with monitors all around her and tubes everywhere. I had just talked to her a couple days before on the phone, and she had been so excited about going to Mexico during April vacation. She was so happy when I had told her that I had bought her a paper suit. When we were saying good-bye, she had said, "I love you." I couldn't believe how much had changed so quickly. I couldn't say a word so I just stood beside her and held her hand.

My first visit to the hospital was an extremely sad time and it's something that I hope I never have to go through again. All of a sudden all of my worries that had seemed so important didn't matter as much. It didn't matter with whom I went to the prom or what I wore to school. I just wanted Kara to get better.

Every time I blow an eyelash over my shoulder and make a wish, it's always that Kara makes a full recovery. Sometimes I'm tempted to wish that I'll do well on my next exam or swim meet but I always push those thoughts out of my mind and think of Kara.

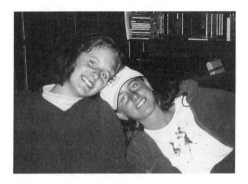

Kara and Guerin tanned by the Maine sun, summer 1996.

CHAPTER 9

Questions with No Answers

ᔕᔕᔕ

What do you say to your daughter when she is seeing her sister lying in a Special Care Unit bed fighting for her life?

Guerin arrived home from Florida on Saturday afternoon and came to the hospital directly from the airport. She looked so cute—all tan with her straight brown hair now sunstreaked, dressed in jean shorts and a blue striped tee shirt.

I met her in the hallway and as we walked into the unit, I tried to give her a quick idea of all of the machines that now surrounded her sister as I prepared her to see Kara. Good preparation is supposed to ease anxiety but I'm not sure that there is any way to prepare for such a sad picture. We entered the room and Guerin went immediately to Kara's side and held her hand and stroked her head. She spoke to her softly and gently cried so that Kara couldn't hear her tears. That picture is frozen in my mind—two sisters, one healthy and one not, and the bond of love between them.

From that first moment, Guerin has always known how to help Kara both physically and emotionally. The mention of Guerin's name has always been able to make Kara smile and brighten up a sad mood. "Guerin" was one of the first words that Kara was able to say as she recovered her speaking abilities in May. I think that perhaps there are no correct words to say; I think it is your strength, your accepting and determined attitudes which are important things to show your daughters, both the healthy and the sick one.

What do you say to your parents when they first see their critically ill granddaughter?

As soon as my parents heard the news of Kara's collapse, they were making plans to fly to Maine from Chicago to help us in any way that they could. My father arrived on Friday night. He is a retired surgeon and was accustomed to hospitals, Special Care Units, ventilators and other accouterments of illness. He was not, however, accustomed to his granddaughter being involved with any of these things. When he first saw Kara, it took his breath away and he cried. I put my arm around him but by then the surgeon in him was already taking over as he told me to make sure that she wasn't getting too much dopamine, as he checked the color and consistency of the urine in her catheter and as he pinched her to see if he could elicit a response. I had asked him to come for one reason. If Kara had no hope for a meaningful recovery, Tom and I together would make the decision to discontinue her life support, but I would need to have my dad say the words "Let her go." There are some words that parents just shouldn't have to say.

The next day my mother came and all that she could do was cry when she saw Kara. Where my mother was a big help to me was at home. As the word of Kara's illness spread throughout the Bath community, our phone was ringing non-stop with words of concern and offers of help and prayers. I was so overwhelmed with the enormity of the situation at the hospital, that I had no ability or energy to deal with the public. Luckily, my mother is a friendly and talkative woman and she fielded all of the telephone conversations beautifully. So much food arrived at our door that I didn't have to cook for four months and my mother carefully recorded who brought what and stored everything in the appropriate spot. She took care of all of the presents and flowers and mail and left me to take care of Kara, Tom, Guerin and myself. She kept my house clean and did all of my wash. It was exactly the help that I needed. My mother was mothering me so that I, in turn, could mother my girls.

What do you say to Kara's fourteen-year-old friends when they come to visit her?

The juxtaposition of Kara's healthy classmates and Kara was a tough emotional experience for me. It was hard for me to see them so healthy and happy and beautiful while Kara lay so helpless in her hospital bed. A week before, she had looked and acted just like them. I was still mourning all of the losses that I was feeling, and I somehsow had to summon the fortitude to explain Kara's condition to these children and console them and their parents.

It was exhausting. And yet I was so proud of them for being strong enough and for caring enough to visit that I didn't want to discourage them. I was caught in this conflict that I had no clue how to resolve. Luckily, the nurses were perceptive about my dilemma and knew what to do. They said simply, "No more visitors!" That was a great help to me and another indication that they were not only treating Kara, but our whole family.

As I got to know other families with sick children at Maine Medical Center, one of the recurring themes was how exhausting it was to talk with people about our children's illnesses. Other people look to the parents for help in understanding the disease process and for consolation and hope. They look to us to cheer them up! It is a paradoxical fact, and one reason that I still choose to go to the grocery store late at night or early in the morning or not at all—to avoid all of those emotionally draining explanations.

How do you know how to act when your life is turned upside down by a sudden and tragic event?

I had no idea how to answer this question but I knew that I had to learn one quickly. Suddenly the answer occurred to me as one day early in Kara's hospitalization I started thinking about Jacqueline Kennedy Onassis. Here was a woman who had suffered through sad, tragic events but always held her head high and walked proudly. She was always gracious, composed and poised through a myriad of public experiences. She kept her life, her children and herself together through situations where others would have crumbled. If she could do it, so could I.

On one especially tough day, Dr. Allan asked me how I was doing. I explained to him my philosophy of pretending to be Jackie O. After that her name became a code word. On the rough days of Kara's unrelenting dystonia when I was trying to be brave and philosophical, he would say, "Very Jackie O." One day he told me that his wife, Ann, was going on a business trip to Arizona. It was a solo business trip in a new job and I said to him, "Very Jackie O.!" as a comment on her independence and spunk. On the day that Kara went to surgery to have her defibrillator implanted, my friend Joanna dropped by our house in the morning with a present and a hug for me. I told her, "I'm Jackie O. today," and she said to me, as I cried on her shoulder, "Today, you don't need to be." But most days I tried hard to live up to Jackie's image.

What do you say to people when they say, "Why are you back at work already?" or "Why are you back at aerobics class already?"

There is an answer to this one and it is easy. You say, "The doctor told me to go back." As long as you say that the doctor told you to do something, people will accept the answer gracefully. When Kara got sick and as the long-term implications of her illness began to register with me, I didn't know how I could possibly leave her to go to work. I visualized myself taking a leave of absence for an undetermined amount of time and spending my days with Kara at the hospital.

One day while Kara was still in the Special Care Unit, Dr. Allan took me aside and asked me what my plans were for returning to work and life. I told him what I was thinking and then he counseled me. He felt that it would be in my best interest and, therefore, in our family's best interest if I went back to my exercise class at the YMCA the next week and back to work at my part-time job in the operating room the week after that. I think that he knew from his experience with other families of brain-injured children what worked best for maintaining good family dynamics. "I can't go back to work," I whined. "I really think that you should think about it. You are in this for a long time and you need to keep part of yourself separate from it," he said.

I thought about it a lot, and in the end I decided that I should heed his advice. He had been down this road before with many other families and I never had. I did go back to my exercise class and to work as he recommended. Although the first few days were tough, there is no doubt in my mind that it was the right decision. My colleagues at work always knew the right words to say and there were even moments of normalcy for me. Both exercise and work have been therapeutic for me in many ways, and I have always been grateful for such good advice. I'm just glad that I listened.

What do you say to people when they say, "You must be so tired of that hour-long car trip to Portland each day"?

That car trip became for me one of the most therapeutic parts of my day. People who understood would say, "The car ride to Portland is one of life's little pleasures." People who didn't understand would say, "Let me keep you company on your long trip to Portland." I used that time in the car to work through my emotions and problems and I relished my time alone. There was no telephone and nobody to disturb me and my thoughts. I would listen to my tapes and find lyrics that reflected my emotional state. The song to which I listened most was the Everly Brother's song "Love Hurts." I must have listened to it over a hundred times, and I cried each time. I knew every chord and every inflection and the words were true to me:

Love hurts, love scars, love wounds and mars
Any heart not tough nor strong enough
To take a lot of pain, take a lot of pain
Love is like a cloud, holds a lot of rain
Love hurts, love hurts

I'm young, I know, but even so
I know a thing or two, I've learned from you
I've really learned a lot, really learned a lot
Love is like a stove, burns you when it's hot
Love hurts, love hurts

Some fools rave of happiness, blissfulness,
togetherness
Some fools fool themselves, I guess
But they're not fooling me.
I know it isn't true, know it isn't true
Love is just a lie, made to make you blue
Love hurts, love hurts

I would make Tom listen to this song and say, "Isn't this true?" and he would tell me I had a depressive personality. But one day, not too long ago, the Everly Brothers were on television singing that song, and Tom cried. You see, it is true.

What do you say to people when they say to you, "I could never be as strong as you are"?

I grew to hate this statement because it involved me having to step out of my role of being the "needy" one and into the role of the "counselor." My answer became rote as I would reply, "I had no choice. We cannot help which cards we are dealt, but how we play them is up to us and I will not fold." I thought it was interesting that I chose this card-playing analogy. I must have some gambling background. Our personalities are composites of our heritage, education, experiences and family, and none of us can share our inner life in sufficient detail to express this. We only know the totality of all of these subtle little things and that is what the world sees as we talk and walk and work and exist together. Somehow the totality of all of my experiences molded me into a resilient person who knew that I would have to look back on Kara's illness in ten or twenty years and be able to say, "I did my best for Kara and for my family."

What do you say when people ask how did this happen to Kara despite all of the prior medical testing and treatment that she had?

Sometimes medicine is just not black and white. People want all diseases and illnesses to fit into neat categories that can easily be diagnosed and treated. Kara had a health problem that just wouldn't clearly identify itself. Despite the fact that she had the best doctors and had all the correct tests, she just wouldn't show us what we needed to see to prevent this from happening.

After much time, thought and many consultations among her physicians, Kara's eventual diagnosis became Long QT syndrome—a heart disorder that can cause fainting, seizures and death. It is hard sometimes to distinguish this disorder from epilepsy. When Kara was in third grade, she was totally worked up both neurologically and cardiologically for fainting spells, and the only norm which was askew was her EEG. She had no symptoms from grades three to eight while she was on Tegretol, an anticonvulsant medication, and only started having problems again after we weaned her from the medication.

Even though the outcome was not the one anyone would have planned, I just don't see anyway that anyone could have done anything differently based on the information that we had at the time. All that we could do now was follow Dr. Hourihan's advice to prevent this from ever happening again and gently prod Kara back to health with medicine, love, patience and hard work.

CHAPTER 10

Kara's Medical History
by Walter Allan, M.D.

လ လ လ

During the first week Kara was in the Special Care Unit
the cardiologists and I were busy trying to figure out why she
had a cardiac arrest. I went back to my chart to review Kara's
history. Reading my written notes and dictations brought back
lots of memories of this young woman. It was easy to recall the
first time I met her. She was one of those kids who even at
eight was very comfortable with adults. The story is everything in neurology and I like to get as much information as
possible from the child. Kids often have insights that are crucial to figuring out what is wrong. Kara would look me straight
in the eye, consider before she answered my question, then
light up the exam room with her smile.

Kara was referred by Dave Enright in Bath because she
had had two unusual episodes of loss of consciousness. The
first had occurred in October 1989 while she was in gym class
rope climbing. She had come down from her climb and felt
what she described as spinning to one side. She put her hand
on the shoulder of a friend and then recalled sliding down to
the floor. The gym teacher reported that Kara was unconscious
and had wet herself. Kara was rushed to the Bath Hospital
emergency room where she seemed fully recovered and had a
normal exam. A few days later she had an EEG that I looked at
and felt was normal and I did not meet her until the second,
more dramatic, episode occurred.

This happened in November 1989. Kara was a competitive swimmer in the Bath YMCA youth program. Maryann
happened to be at the practice and saw the entire event so we
had her story as well as Kara's to go on. Kara jumped from the

block during a practice heat and swam the length of the pool. She made her turn moving somewhat more slowly than when she had started. She then slowed her movements down even further and sank to the bottom of the pool. The other kids had to pull her out. She looked dusky and unconscious at the poolside but was breathing and awoke in seconds.

Kara could recall the beginning of the event. She remembered jumping into the pool and swimming a few strokes. Then she felt like she was, as she put it, "in a dream." She did not recall completing her lap, denied being dizzy or feeling like she was spinning again, and could not remember anything else until she awoke at the side of the pool.

Quite correctly, Dave had sent Kara to one of our pediatric cardiologists, Dick McFaul, for a thorough evaluation. Dick had thought it was serious enough to go beyond the routine ECG and echocardiogram and had done a treadmill study on Kara. She got her heart rate up to greater than two hundred on the treadmill. This was impressive since she started with a resting heart rate of sixty.

Dick described Kara in his note to me as "a competitive eight-year-old with a 'will that exceeds her endurance.'" I was not sure if he was quoting Maryann or describing a type of eight-year-old; in any event it did capture Kara's spirit. He concluded that the episodes were not likely to be cardiac in origin based on the information at hand. But he commented that the lack of a diagnosis was worse than having an explanation in the setting of exercise-related loss of consciousness. So that was why Dave sent her on to me.

Could these episodes be a type of epileptic seizure? Epileptic seizures were certainly a consideration, but it is unusual for seizures to follow strenuous exercise. However, Kara reported feeling as if she were "in a dream" during the last episode and that is one of the attributes of a complex partial seizure. This is a form of seizure that often comes from an epileptic focus in one of the temporal lobes. The temporal lobes are the area of the brain where memories are captured and where vivid dreams are reported by conscious patients undergoing cortical stimulation studies as a part of a neurosurgical procedure. Thus, we repeated Kara's EEG looking for an abnormality that would confirm an epilepsy. This EEG was normal, just as her first one had been, so we decided to watch her for the time being.

In April 1990 she had another episode. Maryann was picking her up from school and Kara was on the playground swinging on a tire. Kara looked odd. Maryann described her as looking "scared" and her pupils were dilated briefly. She acted mildly confused and called, "Mom, Mom..." She then reported that she felt as if she had passed out.

That night Kara said that she had a stomachache and did not eat dinner. After resting she seemed better and hopped up the stairs on one foot. She spoke to Tom for a second in the hall and went to her room. About thirty seconds later Maryann heard heavy breathing coming from Kara's room. She found her face down on the floor having a seizure. The jerking lasted about thirty seconds and Kara awoke within minutes. She did not wet herself. She was seen the next day by Jim Riviello, my partner, who felt the story was quite good for complex partial seizures with secondary generalization, that is, a seizure that would begin in the temporal lobe, spread to involve the rest of the brain and produce a convulsion. He started her on an antiepileptic drug, Tegretol, to prevent them.

I saw Kara in May to check how she was doing and to see what a repeat EEG (her third) would show. Kara was doing fine on the medication and this EEG was also normal. However, the weight of the evidence favored a diagnosis of epilepsy. Because complex partial seizures are sometimes associated with a structural abnormality in the brain, we also did an MRI scan of the brain. This, too, was normal.

My office records showed that Kara did great for the next two years on the Tegretol. There were no more unusual episodes and she continued to be a swimmer and a runner. In June 1992 she had been two years without a spell so we repeated her EEG with the aim of taking her off Tegretol if it were again normal. This time the EEG showed a right frontal sharp wave during sleep. This finding can be a sign of epilepsy and because the episodes had responded so well to treatment and Kara had no side effects, we decided to keep her on the medication.

She continued to do well for two more years and when I saw her in July 1994, she had been four years without an episode of loss of consciousness. She had had two episodes of dizziness during 1993. Both of these had been exercise-related. One occurred after she ran up a flight of stairs and one occurred while she was swimming. But she had not fallen or lost consciousness during either.

When I saw her in the office in July 1994, the EEG no longer showed the right frontal sharp wave. My feeling at that point was Kara had an epilepsy that had resolved as she had matured. This is something that happens in childhood epilepsies. With a normal EEG and no episodes of definite seizures for four years her chances were excellent to remain seizure-free off medication. We decided to wean her from Tegretol over the next month.

Then in August 1994 she had another episode just after she came off Tegretol. She was running uphill when she began to notice lights "coming down" in front of her eyes. She could not recall anything else but a friend reported that Kara had fallen and then had some facial twitches. As she aroused from this episode, she was briefly confused. She was fully recovered by the time the two of them walked back to Kara's house. Maryann called me and Kara was put back on Tegretol. We assumed her epilepsy had not resolved after all.

She did well for awhile but then in February 1995 had a further spell. Once again she was running uphill when it started. Kara said she felt dizzy and saw a blue color prior to falling over backward and having a seizure. Her Tegretol level was below the treatment level so we upped the dose a little.

I saw her in my office for the last time one month before the events of April 7. I remember Kara sitting calmly on my exam table telling me about the blue light she saw before her seizure and smiling her same wonderful smile. Everything seemed fine at that point, and we were all comfortable with Kara on a higher dose of Tegretol. I wrote to Dave Enright, however, that I was not sure Kara had a primary or secondary epilepsy, because things did not exactly add up. Secondary seizures are seizures that occur after some other event—usually a fainting spell. They are not uncommon in teens where fainting is frequent. We usually think of this kind of fainting and the secondary seizure as benign. However, that had not proved to be true in Kara's case. In retrospect, the only clue we had to go on was the association between her spells and exercise.

Thus, as the cardiologists and I reviewed the story and the results of her cardiac evaluation it was obvious that Kara had a primary cardiac arrhythmia that accounted for her arrest on April 7 and likely accounted for many of her spells. The cause of the arrhythmia, however, was not obvious. Kara's heart did not show any signs of a malformation or injury. She did not have any chamber or heart muscle enlargement. Maribeth's and Joel's best guess was Kara had a form of Long QT syndrome without the prolonged QT interval on ECG. To better establish that diagnosis and prevent a cardiac arrest from happening again, or happening to other members of Kara's family, the cardiologists needed to do more tests. This was part of what we did for the next few weeks as we hoped Kara would come out of her coma.

CHAPTER 11

A Roller Coaster Ride

⋴⋺ ⋴⋺ ⋴⋺

When a patient is critically ill, all of the monitoring lines, IVs and various tubes and catheters are inserted quickly, but they are not taken out quickly. One by one, as the patient recovers, these devices are removed, and each removal signals a victory for the patient and the family. Kara had an endotracheal tube which was inserted by the EMTs on the track and was being breathed for by a ventilator. By Sunday, April 9, she had started breathing on her own, and the doctors and nurses were thinking that perhaps she could be extubated. They asked us to leave her room as they made their decision and when we came back into the room, Kara's endotracheal tube had been removed. The head of the bed was positioned so that Kara was sitting, and she still looked just like Sleeping Beauty.

To me, this was a huge milestone because now I knew that she would not be dependent upon a respirator for the rest of her life; it was a positive step in her recovery. I was happy, and it was so nice to see her little face without the tube in her mouth and all of the tape on her cheeks. I felt as if she were the most brilliant child in the world because she was breathing on her own.

On Monday, April 10, Kara smiled for us, and I don't think that I have ever seen a sweeter sight. I was so optimistic, and I thought that we must certainly be on the superhighway to recovery. Dr. Bagwell asked Kara to show her the green elastics on her braces, and Kara complied with the request. I thought that because today she smiled and followed a command, tomorrow she would talk, the next day she would sit up, the next day she would walk, the next day we would go home, and I would say, "See, she is fine." I thought that returning to consciousness from a coma would be similar to wak-ing up from a deep sleep but in slow motion. But we were not on a superhighway; we were on an old, unpaved and bumpy carriage trail. She didn't smile again regularly for about three weeks. She opened her eyes widely for us that Monday but after that she could only open them enough to make little slits. As the days passed, she was able to keep them more widely open and watch us but the recovery was not a smooth progression. It was a series of ups and downs, of good days and rough days, of happiness laced with tears. Dr. Allan would console us by say-ing, "Don't worry. Once she shows a new ability, it is there to stay. You may not see it again for days, but it is there." One of the nurses said to me, "You are in for a roller coaster ride," and she was correct in her prediction.

The most precipitous segment of the roller coaster ride was during the time that Kara was plagued with severe dys-tonic movements that caused her body to go into sudden and severe contortions leaving her sweaty and exhausted and Tom and me distraught. These spasmodic episodes lasted about three weeks. Her heart rate would climb to over one hundred twenty beats per minute during these episodes. It was fright-ening to see her heart working so hard while we still didn't know the cause of her cardiac arrest. As Kara's awareness in-creased she would cry during these episodes. I think that she knew they were happening, that she had no control over them, and they must have been painful. The movements were re-lentless at times, and there was little we could do except to console Kara through them. This was the most difficult por-tion of Kara's recovery for Tom and me. It was painful emo-tionally for us to watch her suffer and to realize that we could never bring her home unless this phase passed.

It was getting hard for me to be hopeful. I wanted to maintain my optimism, but I needed to know that it was still based in reality. I kept telling Kara, "Be brave, Kara, be brave," but it was getting harder for me to be brave. Dr. Allan felt that this stage of dystonia would pass with a little help from time and medication and then he told me something that was the biggest help to me during this phase. "You can be as hopeful as you want. I will tell you when the time for realism arrives." This is called trust.

During this time, Dr. Allan ordered quite a few EEGs for Kara and they all showed improvement, but it was a mystery as to why these dystonic movements continued. At this point Dr. Allan decided that Kara should have an MRI to visualize her brain and show him any possible areas of brain injury. Kara had an MRI when she was in third grade. However, this time she would need to have general anesthesia while she was in the machine because there was no way that she could hold still for an hour. I signed the consent for anesthesia and the anesthesiologist and the resident put her to sleep while I was with her. I don't think that it mattered to Kara because she was not cognizant of much at that point, but it mattered to me a great deal. The exam takes about an hour and I went up to the waiting room where I fell sound asleep on someone else's pillow and the last thought I had was that I hoped that I wasn't going to get lice. I wondered, "How can you possibly be worried about lice when your daughter is having an MRI?" And then I fell asleep.

The waiting room for the Special Care Unit at Maine Medical Center is one of the most interesting places, filled with every human drama. Each family waiting there has a story and each story is dramatic. It is a room filled with a potpourri of people from a potpourri of life experiences and suddenly all of these disparate people were my new best friends. We all shared the ups and downs of our medical progress reports and either rejoiced or consoled depending upon the news. I spent a lot of time in that room observing both strengths and weaknesses of human spirit, and sometimes I saw the greatest strength in the most unlikely people. The nurse from the MRI unit came into the waiting room, woke me, and told me that Kara was back in the Special Care Unit. My hour of rest was over.

The results of the MRI were mixed. The opinions varied depending upon who was reading the MRI. Once again it was a reminder that medicine is sometimes a subjective art of interpretation, but certainly we could feel good that the MRI looked as good as it did and hope it portended a good recovery for Kara.

Still there were reminders that Kara was a fragile cardiac patient who required special skills. When she returned from her MRI, and as I stood at the foot of her bed, both her heart rate and blood pressure dropped, and suddenly she had the attention of all the residents and nurses. Her heart rate was twenty-eight and her systolic blood pressure was in the seventies. Dr. Wayne Sager, a pediatric resident from Montana, was right there. He was a quiet and serious resident who always looked as if he had just slept for twelve hours in his clothes. I had confidence in his ability, though, and I sensed that someday he would make a great pediatrician.

He, I and all the nurses knew that Kara needed some atropine to bring her heart rate and blood pressure back to normal, but first he had to obtain permission from the attending doctor. "It is good that he is checking with Dr. Bagwell," I thought. With Kara's unusual cardiac status, maybe atropine wasn't the correct treatment. But over the telephone, Dr. Bagwell gave her permission for the atropine and a bolus of fluid. Kara's bradycardia and hypotension resolved. It was a reminder that the reason she was in the hospital was a sudden cardiac arrhythmia and the actual cause was as yet undetermined. Obviously there was diagnostic work still to be done.

The main suspect was Long QT syndrome. Since that can be a genetic problem, the cardiologists were interested to see Tom's, Guerin's and my ECGs. The cardiologists had already told us this but then they also sent Dr. Sager to give us the same news. I think that the attending physicians were trying to hone his interpersonal skills by making him deliver unpopular news to parents. He was so apologetic that we had to have ECGs that it would have seemed to anyone observing that he must have been telling us we were all scheduled for open heart surgery the next morning.

Our family was going through so much that I know he felt bad informing us of more potential problems. However, I couldn't resist the obvious joke: "I suppose that next you will

be coming to tell us that we all need cardiac catheterizations."
He assured me that I was being absurd, but the next day he
did tell us that we all did need to have twenty-four-hour ambulatory monitors. "I told you that this was going to escalate.
When are our cardiac catheterizations scheduled?" I asked,
continuing the joke from the day before. I think maybe he was
afraid that I was correct because this time he didn't assure me
that I was being absurd.

At first I thought that all of these tests were an interesting but frivolous technological experience. Then, reality
prevailed and I started to think what the consequences might
be if any of the three of us did have Long QT syndrome. Guerin
was accepted at Providence College in Rhode Island and was
all set to swim on their NCAA Division I swim team. She would
be performing at a high physical level of activity, and we owed
it to her to check her cardiac status. Tom and I had to remain
healthy to help each other and our family through this storm,
and as much as we needed each other, Kara and Guerin needed
us more. It was not a good time for either of us to drop dead,
and so we followed the cardiologists' suggestions and had the
recommended ECGs.

CHAPTER 12

Long QT Syndrome
by Walter Allan, M.D.

৵৵৵

Long QT syndrome is one of the causes of sudden death in adolescents. By sudden death we mean death that occurs out of the blue in a teenager who is apparently healthy. It most frequently occurs during sporting events and is usually attributed to a sudden, unpredictable disturbance in the rhythm of the heart. Sudden death in adolescent athletes is uncommon but always such a shock to their communities that the death of these athletes is well-known and long remembered.

Long QT syndrome is thought to be the cause when sudden death occurs from ventricular fibrillation—a fatal abnormal heart rhythm, or arrhythmia—and no other explanation is found. The syndrome can also become apparent when a young person with fainting or secondary seizures has an ECG as part of their evaluation. It is especially important to look for the syndrome when the fainting or seizures are excercise-related. However, the symptoms can occur during less strenuous activities, upon awakening from sleep, and even when surprised, frightened or angry. Some people discover they have Long QT syndrome when they are being evaluated because a family member has Long QT syndrome. These individuals may have never had fainting or seizures. They are said to have the syndrome because their ECG shows a prolonged QT interval.

Prolongation of the QT interval on the ECG is the major marker for Long QT syndrome. The majority of the QT interval is the time during a single heartbeat when the heart muscle is becoming "recharged" for the next heartbeat. This is called repolarization and follows the phase of heart muscle contraction which actually pumps the blood and is called depolarization. The ECG records the electrical signals from the heart muscle and each wave is labeled as shown.

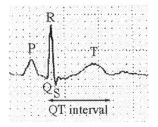

Measuring the distance from the beginning of the Q-wave to the end of the T-wave is the QT interval. By knowing the speed the ECG paper is traveling (usually 25 mm/sec) this measurement can be converted to a time interval. If your heart rate is sixty beats per minute (or one beat per second) the normal QT interval should be less than 0.42 seconds—less than half the time between heart beats. Someone is said to have a long QT interval when this time interval is greater than 0.44 seconds.

There are many difficulties with making this measurement. For instance, the interval varies with the heart rate. In addition, the shape of the T-wave varies among individuals making it difficult to decide what to measure. By correcting the interval for the heart rate (the QTc, for QT corrected) a standardized criteria can be applied. However, what has been learned over time is that not all individuals with the Long QT syndrome have a long QT interval. Thus, it has been suggested that the condition should be called "congenital repolarization syndrome" as that seems to be the real mechanism of the arrhythmia leading to sudden death and would eliminate the contradiction in terms.

Since the syndrome was first described in the 1950s it has become obvious that it is congenital (present at birth) and genetic (inherited). The most common form of inheritance is the autosomal dominant form of Long QT syndrome (Romano-Ward form). Families with this form will have many members that have long QT intervals on ECG. This is because each person has a fifty-fifty chance of having the condition in an autosomal dominant inheritance pattern. Individuals in these families will have symptoms of different severity and some family members with long QT interval will have no symptoms. In addition, there will be family members who must have the syndrome based on the inheritance pattern and who have normal QT intervals! One reason genetic studies of these families was undertaken was to find a gene that marked the disease and to make the diagnosis more certain. This strategy would have great benefit if a gene could be found, given the dire consequences of the condition.

In the past few years there have been important genetic discoveries in Long QT syndrome. These discoveries were made possible in large part by the efforts of Dr. G. Michael Vincent at LDS in Salt Lake City. In the 1970s he became interested in a very large family with a history of sudden death in many members stretching back over generations. This family was descended from two Danish brothers who immigrated to the United States in the nineteenth century. Several members of this family had long QT intervals on their ECGs, and Dr. Vincent became convinced they had the autosomal dominant form of Long QT syndrome.

This disorder was first described in the European medical literature and was little known in the United States at the time. By meticulously searching out this and other large families with sudden death and long QT intervals, Dr. Vincent set the stage for the subsequent discovery of the molecular biology of this condition. By gathering these large family pedigrees enough individuals with a gene for Long QT syndrome were available for the difficult DNA mapping required to establish a genetic link with the condition.

Beginning in 1991 families with Long QT syndrome were discovered to have one of three specific genes that accounted for the syndrome. These genes were found on chromosomes 11 (named LQT1), chromosome 7 (LQT2) and chromosome 3 (LQT3) in different families. In 1995 Dr. Vincent's associate, Dr. Mark Keating, and his molecular biology group at the Howard Hughes Medical Institute of the University of

Utah discovered that these genes produced proteins that were part of heart muscle ion channels. Ion channels are protein pores in the membranes of muscle and nerve cells that allow the cells to rapidly move ions from one side of the membrane to the other. This ion movement produces the electrical properties of depolarization and repolarization that are crucial for heart muscle cell contraction. The ion channels affected by the genes LQT1, LQT2 and LQT3 are all important in heart muscle cell repolarization. Since the length of the QT interval mostly represents repolarization of the heart as a unit, their discovery fit the theory that problems with heart muscle cell repolarization were the cause of Long QT syndrome.

Thus, the story of Long QT syndrome is becoming clearer as to what really happens to produce the long QT interval (the abnormal ion channels) and who is at risk for sudden death (family members with the actual gene). The pieces of the puzzle still missing are the reason that some people with the gene will and some will not have severe ventricular arrhythmias and what other genes are involved. Researchers know that there must be more than three genes that can produce Long QT syndrome since a French group has recently mapped another gene (LQT4 on chromosome 4). Some families with Long QT syndrome do not have any of these four genes.

Much of this information became known to our group of physicians while Kara was at Maine Medical Center, and eventually she and her family were put in contact with Dr. Keating's lab. But that is getting ahead of the story. As it became apparent that Kara probably had Long QT syndrome, it was important to protect her from another event. Her ECG showed normal QTc intervals most of the time, but some intervals were up to 0.50 seconds in length. Thus, she was kept on constant ECG monitoring until the cardiologists came up with an appropriate solution. In the first week we were not sure if Kara would make a meaningful recovery so monitoring alone seemed best. A bigger problem was to be sure the rest of the Anglim family was not at risk.

The Anglims are all athletes. Tom runs miles everyday

at lunch. Maryann does aerobics three times a week. Guerin, as a high school senior, was voted "Swimmer of the Year" for 1995 in Maine's Class B and won the state 100-yard backstroke event. None of them had any recent problems, but because of the dominant inheritance pattern of Long QT syndrome they needed to have their ECGs checked. Tom's and Guerin's looked fine, but Maryann's had a 0.49 QTc and a U-wave (see below). These findings were enough to make our cardiologists monitor the three of them with ambulatory ECG recorders. This is a tape recorder-sized ECG machine with miniature chest leads that records heart beats constantly while worn. This test failed to show any arrhythmia in Tom, Guerin or Maryann, and Maryann's further evaluation was put off given all the other problems the Anglims were facing.

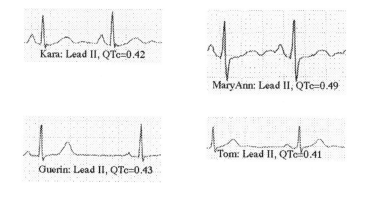

Kara: Lead II, QTc=0.42

MaryAnn: Lead II, QTc=0.49

Guerin: Lead II, QTc=0.43

Tom: Lead II, QTc=0.41

CHAPTER 13

Kara's MRI Scan
by Walter Allan, M.D.

৵ ৵ ৵

Kara's neurological status after the first week of her hospitalization was a problem. She had at first improved quickly. By the evening of April 7 the nurses noted she was spontaneously opening her eyes. This marked the official end of her coma. Because of this I was able to give the Anglims good news when we met later that first night.

The system I use to try to predict outcome gives the best statistical outlook to patients with an examination that includes eye opening by six hours. However, that estimate is still in the range of only about a fifty percent chance for a good recovery. These estimates come from a paper by D. E. Levy and other neurologists at Cornell Medical Center in New York. They examined comatose patients admitted after cardiac arrest at six hours and then daily for two weeks. They compared what they saw on the exam with the patient's outcome at one year and constructed tables for neurologists to use as guides. This study is the best source of information I know of as it is based on two hundred ten such patients. This is more than any other study of outcome in anoxic coma, that is, coma caused by lack of oxygen. If Kara was going to remain in the most favorable category for recovery, she should have been following commands by a week. She was not.

When I examined Kara each day I would start by calling her name a few times to see if she would arouse and open her eyes. I would then try to get her to follow my face or turn toward me by continuing to call her name. By a week she was able to do this consistently. Next I would try to get her to follow commands in response to the words I was saying. These

58

would be fairly simple things, such as, "close your eyes," "stick out your tongue," "open your hand," "wiggle your toes." Kara could not or would not do these things.

There were other disturbing signs as well. Out of the blue Kara would suddenly become opisthotonic. This is a very disturbing dystonic movement in which the patient arches to an extreme degree. Kara would grit her teeth, extend her legs, point her toes, pull her flexed arms tightly against her chest with her hands fisted and arch her trunk throwing her head back. These episodes were quite difficult for the family and the nurses to watch. She would hold this position for ten to fifteen seconds, often sweating profusely. Then she would relax briefly before it would start over again. We could not be sure if we were setting these episodes off by something we were doing to her or not. Decreasing stimulation by lowering the lights and not touching her did not seem to make these episodes better. Everyone wanted them to stop.

I discussed medications with some of my colleagues and tried putting Kara on lorazepam (a minor tranquilizer and anticonvulsant) to see if we could diminish the episodes. As part of discussing Kara's episodes with other neurologists the question of her prognosis would come up. They were hard pressed to be optimistic mainly because these opisthotonic episodes were still persisting at a week after her cardiac arrest.

However, despite these episodes and not following direct commands, Kara was doing some very positive things that put her outside the classification system devised by Levy. At least that was my feeling. For instance, she would have periods of alertness in which she would survey her surroundings, and she made good eye contact with her parents and her friends. When I would get her into the sitting position with her legs over the side of the bed, she could lift her head and look at me making little adjustments in her trunk to right herself. She even grabbed the bed's side rail at around this time to position herself and looked as if she were attempting to sit up spontaneously. Because of these abilities I remained cautiously optimistic with the Anglims.

To get a better idea if my optimism was appropriate I sent an e-mail message to my good friend Steve Rothman at Washington University in St. Louis. Steve and I trained together and he had gone on to become the chief of our training program in child neurology at St. Louis Children's Hospital, as well as a world renowned researcher in neuronal cell death. His opinion would carry weight and I knew he would have heard the latest about neurologic outcome after anoxia. My message described Kara's story and her exam. I asked him what he thought about possible areas of damage and what he thought the outlook was.

Steve wrote back, "The patient you described is my nightmare, in that I am always worried that some kid I say has seizures will turn out to have an arrhythmia." He mentioned the Levy article as the one he used for prognosis and noted the fact that following commands at one week was the most important sign of good outcome. He went on to suggest Kara's areas of damage might be in the hippocampus and cortex.

Steve's note was both good and bad. I could feel confident that I knew all there was to know as far as the neurologic literature on outcome was concerned. However, significant damage in the hippocampus meant she might recover to a state of total amnesia. This is a horrible state in which the person is unable to learn anything new. Significant cortical damage could result in any of a number of problems from paralysis to a mindless conscious state in which she would not be in touch even with her past memories and not recognize her family and friends. Of course, it was implied in my discussions with the family that something as horrible as this was possible. However, we did not talk openly about such dire consequences. This is because there was no certain way to know that such a future lay ahead for Kara. There was nothing we could do to prevent it even if it did.

That was the setting in which we decided to do magnetic resonance imaging (MRI). MRI scans became available in the late 1980s. By using a very intense magnetic field and sophisticated computer analysis it is possible to produce images of the brain that are of remarkable detail. In Kara's case we could detect even minor areas of damage which would hope-fully tell us more about her outlook. I was reluctant to do an MRI earlier in Kara's hospitalization because two to three days are required for injury to become apparent. In addition, be-cause of Kara's arching she would have to have general anes-thesia to be still enough to get the images. This might present some danger to her heart. Since she had been at Maine Medi-cal Center, we had seen no signs of an arrhythmia and she had been on continuous monitoring.

On the eleventh hospital day she had the hour-long MRI scan under general anesthesia. Everything went well and technically good images were obtained. However, when she returned to the Special Care Unit she suddenly dropped her heart rate to twenty-eight beats per minute and had to be given atropine to get her rate back to normal. This event reminded us of how unstable her cardiac status was and how careful we needed to be to guard her against another cardiac arrest.

The MRI images were a surprise. I could not see any lesions when I looked the study over alone. Our neuroradiologists debated whether or not she might have some injury in the substantia nigra—the area that degenerates in Parkinsonism. But they, too, were amazed at how little seemed to be wrong with the images. Usually we are in the position of seeing large areas of abnormality in the MRI images and not knowing if they will be permanent or not. After a brain injury there might be areas of brain swelling that are injured but able to recover as well as permanently injured areas. Both of these types of brain swelling show up easily. So Kara's scan was de-cidedly different from what we expected.

I sent copies to Steve to review with the chief of neuroradiology at Washington University. He did not think the substantia nigra was injured and saw subtle changes in the insula—a part of the temporal lobes of the brain. But he and Steve were also amazed at how little they saw. This was good for Kara and supported my optimism with the Anglims. We were going to have to base our estimate of how Kara would do on her day-to-day exam. Basically we were saying we would just have to wait and see.

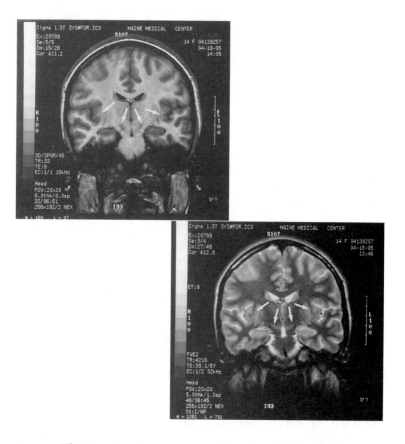

The images above are complementary coronal images in the same plane made with different imaging parameters so that pathologic features will be demonstrated. The image on the left is called "T-1" weighted and the image on the right is called "T-2" weighted. Images in the coronal plane are oriented so that if you were able to look directly through a face millimeter by millimeter, this is the view of the brain you would see. Kara's right hemisphere is on the left side of each picture. The middle two arrows in each picture point to the substantia nigra. It appears to be too dark on the T-1 image and too bright on the T-2 image, according to the neuroradiologist at Maine Medical Center. The lateral two arrows in each picture point to the insula of each hemisphere. Very subtle changes are seen there according to the neuroradiologist at Washington University in St. Louis.

CHAPTER 14

Decisions

৩ ৩ ৩

Even though a routine may be a difficult one, it is still a routine and there is a comfort in understanding the patterns and rhythms of the day. The Special Care Unit had become a routine way of life for me, and I was content to exist in its world. I knew what to expect from the nurses, doctors and residents, and I knew what they expected of me. I knew how much care they would let me do for Kara and what they wanted to do themselves. I knew a little about each of their personalities and lives and they were learning about me. But Kara was getting better and was no longer in need of their special brand of care and it was time for her to make room in the unit for someone who did.

Because of her still unstable cardiac condition, she needed to be transferred to a cardiology unit where her heart could be monitored constantly and where the nursing staff was accustomed to caring for cardiac patients. The decision about where to transfer Kara was difficult. The nurses would be caring not only for a cardiac patient, but also a pediatric patient who happened to have both neurologic and rehabilitative needs. She was a complex patient who would push the limits of any nurse's knowledge and skill.

Finally, after eleven days in the Special Care Unit, it was decided that Kara would be transferred to R-9, a step-down cardiac unit, where Kara would be on telemetry which is a method of constant cardiac monitoring using radio signals. I was anxious about this move because I was afraid of the unknown; there would be new personalities, new standards of care, new routines, new rules, new everything. I am sure that the nurses were anxious, too; Kara was a sick little girl who needed a lot of physical and medical care and her story must have left their emotions raw. With trepidation and as much optimism as I could muster, Kara and I made the long trip down the hall and up nine floors in the elevator to R-9 and a new chapter of Kara's hospitalization.

The code of hospital care is that the sickest patients are always put in the room directly across from the nursing station and that is exactly where Kara went. I was trying to have a good attitude about this new nursing unit, but the first shock was that Kara had a roommate. "Well, that is okay," I said to myself. "We can get along with most anyone." But the roommate turned out to be an older woman who kept the television volume up, belched loudly with regularity and insisted on having the curtain drawn between the two beds. Kara's bed was on the side of the room away from the window, and I didn't see how I was going to survive.

She was still dystonic, and when she had the spasms which made her back arch and legs extend, Tom and I could often help break their cycle if we could urge her to relax and bend her head forward. Doing this took a lot of physical and emotional strength, and we needed space in which to do this. We had none.

By this time, Tom and I had developed the routine where I would be with Kara during the day, and he would come to the hospital after his work day, staying with her until she fell asleep in the evening. Once he got to the hospital, we talked for a while and caught up on each other's day, and then I came home to be Guerin's mom for the evening. When he came to the hospital that day, I couldn't even talk. I think he walked in and I walked out. That day I left the hospital discouraged, tearful and filled with self-pity, wondering how my life could be any worse.

The problem must have been obvious to the nurses because when I arrived the next morning, Kara's roommate was gone. The nurses and I moved Kara's bed over to the window, turned on the MTV station for her and decorated the room with cards and posters. My mood improved. The nurses on R-9 had Kara as a patient through an extremely difficult segment of her recovery, and they worked hard to understand her medical problems and keep her safe and comfortable.

During this stage of her hospitalization Kara was in an almost constant state of movement due to the dystonia and restlessness. She would move so much that she rubbed her toes, elbows and knees raw on the sheets and so the nurses arranged for Kara to have a special air bed with Gortex sheets. She had to be watched closely because she would move with such strength and persistence that she could flip herself out of the bed. She became so sweaty that we were constantly reapplying the ECG stickers as they fell off her. It took two people to bathe her, one person to pry up her arms and the other person to wash underneath them. She slept little during this phase and she kept the nurses, Tom and me busy.

On April 25, I wrote this in my journal:

> I should have started this sooner but I couldn't because Kara keeps me so unbelievably busy when I'm here. Her dystonia is unrelenting at times and hard for me to watch but also I think hard for her to bear. She seems to know that she cannot control her muscles and that makes her cry and be scared. It is so pitiful to watch.
>
> This is so different than I thought it would be. I thought that there would be quiet moments when I could read to her and talk gently to her...

That is the end of my entry that day. Obviously the last paragraph I wrote was true.

But there were bright moments, too. In late April, Kara became increasingly more able to follow commands and we could easily make her smile. She could delight us by touching her tongue to her nose when we asked her. The speech therapist was able to get Kara to enjoy sucking on a lollipop. The occupational and physical therapists were able to get Kara to kick a soccer ball and she was starting to walk, although she still needed a great deal of support for this task. She started using the toilet. She started eating a little bit of applesauce and jello although her main source of nutrition was the feeding through her nasogastric tube.

Tom, Guerin and I could get her up in a wheelchair and leave the confines of her room and cruise around R-9. We couldn't leave the telemetric field so we couldn't go off of the unit, and we must have walked and wheeled Kara around the circumference of that floor at least a million times. Neurologically she was getting better, but it was during Kara's stay in this cardiology unit that we began to deal with the questions of how to handle her long-term nutritional and cardiac needs.

I had a hard time accepting the inevitability of a gastrostomy feeding tube semipermanently inserted in Kara's stomach. To me it acknowledged the fact that her recovery would be slow and laborious, and I fought the thought of it for awhile. I was sure that I could feed her enough jello, soup and pudding to avoid this dreaded feeding tube. Slowly I came to realize that excellent nutrition was a strong component of Kara's recovery and that I couldn't let my feelings come in the way of her future health.

Because of Kara's dystonia it was obvious that she could not take sufficient calories by mouth to keep up with her demands. Even though she spent most of her time in bed at this stage, her caloric demands were great. For instance, she was not sleeping well, moving and thrashing through most of the night. In addition, during her dystonic episodes, her heart rate would climb to one hundred forty and she would sweat excessively. In order to get better, she needed to have a reliable source of calories for an extended period of time. The only solution to this problem was a gastrostomy tube. I had to accept it as a positive step, and my attitude changed just in time as the surgeons and their nurses began to visit us in Kara's room with their plans and advice.

Once again a nurse came to my psychiatric aid. Nancy Tkasc, the pediatric surgeons' nurse, had the awesome task of serving as the liaison between the surgeons and their patients and families. She told me not to feel bad about the tube, that in time Kara's tube would come out and that many of their patients just used it at night time for what they called "recreational feeding" to give their nutritional needs a boost and help with their healing process. Through the course of Kara's hospitalization, I realized what a lifesaver the gastrostomy tube was. On those days when Kara wouldn't or couldn't eat well, we always had the tube feedings to rely upon for her caloric needs. I started fantasizing about how much time could be saved if our whole family had feeding tubes. There would be no more grocery shopping, no more cooking or dish washing and with all of our spare time we could become great philanthropists or philosophers or see every old movie that we always wanted to view but for which we never had time. If only we all had feeding tubes, this would all be possible.

It was easier to accept the inevitability of the combination pacemaker/defibrillator device than the feeding tube. As Dr. Cutler's nurse told me, "Once you have a patient who experiences ventricular fibrillation, you have two choices: to put a defibrillator in the patient or to put a defibrillator in the patient." These black and white choices make decisions easy. So, together Tom and I took a deep breath and said "yes" to both the gastrostomy feeding tube and the cardiac device, an implantable cardiac defibrillator (ICD).

It was while Kara was a patient on cardiology that I met our favorite resident, Yvonne. She was so beautiful that I always felt as if I were staring at her. She was tall, exotic-looking with long black hair down to her waist. I kept trying to figure out what her ethnic origins were. "She could be South American," I thought, "or maybe Samoan, or maybe Hawaiian." I finally decided that she was Hawaiian, but one day I asked Dr. Allan what nationality she was. The answer was Native American from New Mexico. I admired her so much and during Kara's care, we became "hospital" friends. She told me that she had a little boy who looked just like her husband. Someday I hope that she will have a little girl who looks just like her. Her goal was to become a pediatric psychiatrist and now she was on her pediatric neurology rotation and Kara became her patient. Yvonne was a good clinician, and brought a psychosocial dimension to Kara's treatment by reminding us that despite Kara's condition she was a fourteen-year-old girl who still had all the emotions and needs of any adolescent.

One day she told me that she was going on a short vacation so she wouldn't be seeing us for a few days. When I asked her where she was going, she said, "New Mexico." I thought that she was probably just going to visit her family and friends for a few days, but I later found out that she went to give the commencement address at her high school. She was the only person from her high school who had ever gone on to become a physician. She was an incredible woman, not only because she was a doctor, but also because she was so quietly proud. I hope that those graduates listened closely to her speech because there was a lot to learn from Yvonne. To me, she was another example of our bittersweet hospital experiences; yes, it was sad that Kara was seriously ill and having a gastrostomy tube and a defibrillator inserted and I would have given anything to have two healthy daughters, but it was a privilege for all of our family to meet someone with Yvonne's personality and abilities. I hope that my daughters grow up to be just like her.

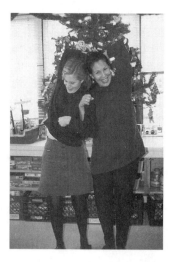

*Kara clowning with Dr. Yvonne at Christmas 1996
on Pediatrics.*

CHAPTER 15

Acronyms

Dr. Allen Browne was the pediatric surgeon who was going to insert Kara's gastrostomy feeding tube April 25. Everyone was referring to the tube by its abbreviation PEG, percutaneous gastrostomy tube. Normally, the patient is merely sedated, but because Kara could not hold still of her own volition, she was going to have general anesthesia. Also, she needed a fluoroscopic stomach X-ray study to make sure that she didn't have a condition known as reflux in which the stomach contents would flow up into the esophagus instead of down into the small intestines. If a patient does have reflux, the PEG can still be inserted, only lower in the gastrointestinal tract.

The X-ray was scheduled for 2:00 p.m. on a day I was working, but I was able to get away early to be with Kara. I couldn't imagine how she was going to lie still enough for a radiologist to get an accurate X-ray, but I knew it would help if I could talk to her, position her and break any dystonic episodes that might occur while she was under fluoroscopy. Luckily, Linda had decided to come and visit with Kara and me at the hospital that afternoon; if she had known the workout that she was gong to get and the amount of radiation that she was going to be exposed to that day, she probably would have rescheduled her visit.

Together Linda, Kara, a nurse and I all went down to the X-ray department through a long hallway painted with gigantic bright flowers. Linda and I wondered what Kara thought about those huge flowers as we wheeled her past them. We decided that she must have felt as if she were Alice in Wonderland, when Alice had made herself little and was amongst the flowers in the garden. Those flowers served their purpose well;

69

they distracted us for a few minutes, giving us a momentary respite from the reality of the hospital.

Once we arrived, the plan was to lift Kara into the fluoroscopy machine where Dr. Charlie Grimes, the radiologist, would inject the dye into Kara's nasogastric tube. Then he would take the X-rays as we flipped Kara from side to side while he watched and recorded how Kara's stomach emptied. Linda and I just looked at each other and the look said, "How the hell is this ever going to work?" Linda and I both donned lead aprons. We continually talked and soothed Kara and before we knew it, we were both halfway inside the X-ray machine with her. The radiologist would say, "Turn her on her right side," and then, "Turn her on her left side," and then, "Turn her on her back," as he would take the X-ray.

When he was finished, he came out to tell us that her study looked normal and I asked him, "How did Linda's hands look?" She has arthritis in her fingers and he must have had a complete radiographic study of both our hands. He replied, "Well, I didn't notice your hands, but I could see that you have big hearts." It was a sweet thing to say and it made Linda and me smile. I think that Dr. Grimes must have a big heart, too, because he took the time to notice and comment. We just thought that we were doing what was right but he saw something more.

As the day for the PEG insertion neared, I told Tom that since it was more a procedure than a surgery, he didn't need to take time off from his dental practice and that I could handle it alone. On the afternoon of the procedure, two orderlies came up from surgery to put Kara on a stretcher and take her down to the operating room suite. I started getting unreasonably nervous. They were here to take my daughter away from me, and they looked as if they hadn't had a shave or shower in a week. The words "escaped convicts" came to my mind. We all rode on the elevator down many floors to the operating room where nurses and doctors greeted us and quickly took Kara away from me. I hastily kissed her and then she was gone. One nurse called out to me as they went through the doors to the operating room, "Don't worry, we will take good care of her." As an operating room nurse myself, I had said those same words to parents and family members so many times. Now I knew for certain how important those words were. The doors shut behind Kara and her entourage, and I was left all alone hoping that they were going to put a PEG in and not take her tonsils out. I had to trust their skill and expertise and I did, but I realized that I had made a mistake when I told Tom that I could handle it alone. I needed his hand to hold.

During the hour that Kara was in the operating room, Dr. Browne passed an EGD (esophago-gastro-duodeno) scope through her mouth and into her stomach. Her stomach was inflated with air to enlarge it. Dr. Browne then looked at Kara's belly to see the light on the end of the scope through her abdominal wall. Using a large gauge needle, he punctured her skin and inserted the needle into her stomach. A long wire was then passed through the needle and caught using the scope so that it could be pulled up and out Kara's mouth leaving the other end protruding out the abdominal wound. The PEG was attached to the wire and pulled back down through her esophagus into the stomach and out through the needle hole. This created a tight fit for the tube. A flange on the stomach side pulled the stomach wall up against the skin. For a few days there would be some leaking, but then the inflammatory response would create a semipermanent seal for the gastrostomy tube. Because of the relatively benign nature of this surgery, Kara could begin using the tube for feeding within a day. Later when I told Tom the details about this procedure, he said in his usual droll manner, "Do not attempt this procedure at home."

As Kara slept off the sedation that had been given to her in the operating room, she looked as peaceful and relaxed as I had seen her look in weeks. The dystonia was gone. As the anesthesia wore off, however, the dystonia returned as severely as ever and talking to her and flexing her head forward were of no help in breaking the spasms. Just at this time, Dr. Bagwell stopped by for an unofficial visit which quickly became official. She assessed the problem as one driven by pain and ordered some morphine to be given intravenously. The morphine helped Kara greatly through the night but it was the start of an unsettled week medically for Kara. Her restlessness was constant and she was upset all of the time. Since Kara couldn't speak and tell us what the problem was, it was difficult for the doctors and nurses to determine the cause. It was another time of heartbreak where the temptation to despair loomed ever present for me. Finally it became apparent that Kara had pneumonia. The symptoms of restlessness, crying and dystonia started to diminish once the pneumonia began to resolve itself with the help of antibiotics.

Tom and I were just recovering from this difficult week when the doctors determined that it was time for Kara to get her ICD implanted. This device both paces the heart when the rate falls below a preset number of beats per minute and delivers an electrical shock to the heart to restore a normal rhythm when a tachyarrhythmia has occurred. Now we were talking to the cardiac clinical nurse specialist, Deb Courtney. Deb is a wonderfully knowledgeable and friendly woman who was able to show us the actual device and to give us an idea how it worked and how it would affect Kara's life. Once again, I knew that if Tom and I accepted the ICD as a part of who and what our family now was, that Kara and Guerin would, too. It is easy to be mature when there is no other choice. Basically Deb told us that Kara would be able to do any physical activity that she was capable of but that contact sports were definitely out of the question. The fragile part of an ICD are the wires which connect it to the heart and constant pummeling of them could cause them to break. So soccer would not be a part of Kara's life anymore. It seemed a small price to pay for such a miraculous little device.

The surgery was scheduled for Monday May 8 with both Dr. Reed Quinn, the pediatric cardiac surgeon, and Dr. Cutler. Dr. Quinn would make the "pocket" for the device in Kara's lower left abdomen and make the incision in her left clavicular area for the wires. Dr. Cutler would thread the wires through Kara's subclavian vein into her right ventricle and her superior vena cava, place the leads where he wanted them, set their electrical parameters and then let them work their magic.

During the surgery, Dr. Cutler would put Kara in ventricular fibrillation twice and make sure that the device defibrillated her appropriately and returned her heartbeat to a normal sinus rhythm. "These guys have nerves of steel," I thought.

Dr. Quinn came to Kara's room to have me sign the consent the Friday before the surgery. It was during the day, so it was my shift. I have checked so many surgical consents in my career as an operating room nurse and never in my wildest imagination did I ever dream that I would be signing a consent for our daughter to have a defibrillator/pacemaker inserted. Dr. Quinn is a tall and taciturn Irish-looking man; he resembled one of my Irish cousins. He carefully explained to me his role in Kara's surgery and said that I was under no obligation to sign the consent. "For example," he said, "if you don't like my tie, you don't have to sign." But, I liked his red tie, and I liked him and we knew that this was the correct treatment for Kara, so I signed. It was easier than I thought it would be.

Once again orderlies came to pick up Kara for surgery. This time Tom was with me and it was an easier wait because he was there. Again they briskly wheeled her into surgery and there was only time for the briefest of farewells. That was probably just as well because too much time would have allowed the reality of our situation to take hold and tears would have followed. Kara didn't need to see us cry; she needed to see us act bravely, as if getting a defibrillator implanted was a normal and every day occurrence.

Just as Tom and I were about to get maudlin, Linda and her daughter Michelle arrived and insisted that we all go out to lunch. The surgery was scheduled to take three hours so we let the nurses know where we were going and reluctantly I went out to lunch. "This is too weird," I thought. "How can you eat lunch while your daughter is having surgery?" I really preferred to stay at the hospital and sit and worry, but when I am feeling adrift and someone I know and respect gives me advice, I feel as if I should listen because I know my thinking must be muddled.

We came back to the hospital after two hours, just in time to see Dr. Cutler who had jogged up nine flights of stairs to tell us that the surgery had gone well, the leads were where he wanted them and the device had defibrillated appropriately when he had put Kara in ventricular fibrillation. How do you thank someone who has just guided your daughter through something like this? There are no other words but "thank you," and they seemed pitifully inadequate. I hope he knew how grateful we were. I knew from my own experience as an operating room nurse that two hours to put a complicated patient to sleep and place two leads and an ICD was a short time; the surgery must, indeed, have gone well.

The recovery room was atypically slow that afternoon, and the nurses allowed Tom, Linda, Michelle and me to sit quietly by Kara while she awoke. This time they gave her plenty of fentanyl, a narcotic pain reliever, and that was the beginning of a smoother postoperative course for Kara, Tom and me. I felt relieved knowing that her cardiac problem was controlled, which is the most that we could hope for since a cure for Long QT syndrome is not possible at this time. Now with that behind us, we could concentrate on her neurologic and rehabilitative recovery.

CHAPTER 16

Kara's Defibrillator
by Walter Allan, M.D.

❧ ❧ ❧

The decision to surgically place an ICD in Kara was a difficult one. It took input from our cardiologists and Kara herself. Joel Cutler, our cardiac electrophysiologist, first saw Kara on her third hospital day. The question for him at that time was what had caused Kara's episode of ventricular fibrillation and what should be done about it. He expected to see a comatose fourteen-year-old who either would not survive or would not survive in any meaningful way. This is the usual result of an out-of-hospital cardiac arrest. Thus, because the outlook is usually so bleak he really thought his role was going to be simply to make a diagnosis. After reviewing the chart and discussing Kara's story with Maribeth Hourihan, the pediatric cardiologist, he was convinced Kara had Long QT syndrome. This had major implications for the family and planning their evaluation was going to be his focus. However, Joel said it took him five minutes of talking with Maryann to decide he was also going to have to put a defibrillator in Kara. It was obvious she was going to survive and just as obvious that Maryann's personality was such that she would optimize whatever recovery Kara made and would expect her daughter to be protected.

One of the factors that made that decision easier for Joel was the nature of implantable defibrillators. In the year prior to Kara's event a new ICD had become available. This device had gone from a bulky oversized item not suited for use in the pediatric population to the miniaturized form he was now using. The tiny ICD available for Kara was a battery-operated, computerized electronic device that could sense her cardiac rhythm, pace her heart if the rate fell below a set limit and defibrillate her if ventricular fibrillation ever recurred.

And the method of implanting an ICD had become easier. The method in 1995 was percutaneous, through the skin—much the same way he did a cardiac catheterization. Prior to this development, it had required a sternal-splitting thoracotomy, or opening the patient's chest. That would have meant a major operation for Kara, and she would not be in any shape for that to be done for a very long time. However, using the percutaneous approach, the ICD's two heart leads would be inserted through the subclavian vein under her clavicle. They could then be directed into position in her right ventricle and her superior vena cava. The leads would be connected to the device nestled under her skin on her lower abdomen. This could be done with little danger to Kara. The lead in the ventricle is a tripolar lead that does the sensing and pacing. It also has a long coil that is used to deliver the shock that could defibrillate the heart. The lead in the superior vena cava is also a coil and is, in effect, the other paddle in administering a defibrillating countershock—the step that had saved her life on April 7, 1995.

After his first meeting with Maryann, the question for Joel became when should the ICD be implanted. The answer lay with Kara. First she would have to improve enough so that leaving the hospital was a reasonable idea. My first thought that this was going to happen came at the end of the second week of her hospitalization. It involved learning more about Tom as well as a change in Kara's condition.

Kara was continuing to have severe dystonic movements that consisted of flexing her arms to her chest, extending her legs and arching her back. She would look very uncomfortable and moan or cry during these episodes. Tom and Maryann found they could stop her posturing by talking to her. Kara would seem to stop and attend to their voices and faces. She also would stop if you flexed her neck forward during an episode. This became a routine with Tom and me.

When I was seeing Kara in the evening at the end of my hospital rounds Tom would be on duty. Kara often thrashed about and postured as Tom and I were talking. He reached over the rail of her bed, in midsentence, and gently but firmly flexed her neck forward. Kara quieted and relaxed for several minutes. When it happened again and she was closer to my side of the bed, I flexed her neck forward with the same result, and our conversation would continue without a hitch. The nonchalance that Tom brought to this act showed me that he, like Maryann, was going to make this situation turn out the best it could for their family, no matter what Kara's eventual neurologic function. This was a solid family that was going to solve whatever problems came their way, together and intact.

But then there was Kara herself. One morning, during her third week in the hospital, when I came by to check on her, I saw her smile at me as I came to her bedside. It was a smile I knew well from Kara's visits to my office, the smile that lit up the room. She still could not talk at this point in her recovery. Thus we had no way of knowing what she was thinking. That smile convinced me she had her personality intact. My view was that she was okay inside all that dystonic posturing. This is the sort of thing families will tell you about their neurologically damaged child. I am as guilty as the next neurologist of rolling my eyes when I hear this. We mark it down to wishful thinking. But I knew Kara and I knew that smile.

This had never happened to me before in my twenty years in practice. I had never had the experience of knowing the child as well as I knew Kara before a terrible event such as this. I could see what the Anglims could see. She did attend to them in a way that was more than mindless vigilance. Of all the things that happen after brain injury, change in personality is the worst. All too often after generalized brain injury the individual's reaction to family, friends and to situations is so drastically changed that families say they are "not the same person." This can so alter the patient's acceptance back into the family that the rehabilitation ultimately fails. Despite the cognitive skills, and the movement quality, if the patient's personality is altered the end result can be a disaster. I knew on April 21 that was not going to be Kara's fate.

For Kara to get to the next stage in her recovery she needed to move to the pediatric floor. She had to come off telemetry and the only way for her to do that safely was to have her ICD implanted. Joel, with the help of the pediatric cardiac surgeon, did this in early May. In order to know that the device worked correctly he had to pace the heart, record from the device's memory and then induce ventricular fibrillation and defibrillate her heart. The ICD works by sensing when a very rapid heart rate occurs. It then charges its capacitors and delivers a shock. Joel had to make sure that the shock needed to defibrillate Kara was within the limit of the device. He chose a shock that was about two-thirds of the maximum and it worked in the operating room without a hitch. Hopefully, this would fulfill Maribeth Hourihan's promise to the Anglims that Kara would never have a cardiac arrest again.

CHAPTER 17

The Bad, Bad Bed

⋙ ⋙ ⋙

Kara's defibrillator/pacemaker was put in May 8. Now that we had her cardiac status protected, it was time to concentrate on improving her cognitive and physical skills in an environment where the staff was accustomed to dealing with adolescents who were sick medically as well as physically challenged—The Pediatric Unit.

This time transferring Kara from one nursing unit to another went amazingly well. Since Dr. Allan is a pediatric neurologist, his hospitalized patients often ended up on the Pediatric Unit, and he had a warm rapport with the pediatric nurses and this rapport served his patients well. He had the entire staff prepared for Kara's arrival—they knew her story and special needs. Lisa Jackson, the assistant head nurse, and some of her nursing staff had attended the weekly patient care conferences on the cardiology unit, and they understood every detail of Kara's status.

Tom and I were looking forward to Kara's transfer because to us moving to pediatrics meant freedom from telemetry. While Kara was a patient on cardiology, she had to remain within the confines of the telemetric field which meant that we could never leave the ninth floor with Kara. The ninth floor at Maine Medical Center is a great place with views of the White Mountains and the Portland Sea Dogs' baseball field, but we were ready for more than this. We were ready for the hospital cafeteria, the Maine Mall, the movies, the Mexican restaurant near-by and walks on the promenade. Kara still had to go in a wheelchair to these places but at least she could go out in the fresh air and sunshine now.

I did miss the nurses on cardiology after our move. They had been Kara's nurses through the roughest stages of

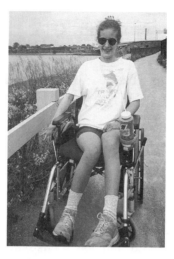

Kara on a wheelchair outing around the Back Cove in Portland, June 1995.

Kara's dystonia and had worked hard to understand and help both her and us through this stage of Kara's sleepless nights and muscle spasms. Many of them shared the stories of their lives with me; that helped me a lot. Some of them had made it through difficult medical situations with their own children and were now happy and functioning people, filled with great compassion. I was a member in their club now, and I would feel proud if I could only be like them. Some of them would come into Kara's room early in the mornings before I arrived at the hospital and take their coffee breaks with Kara as they watched MTV together. They would take the time to French-braid Kara's hair and dress her in cute matching shorts and tee shirts. They never dwelled on what Kara couldn't do and would joyfully report to Tom and me every new function that they observed returning to our daughter. But now it was time to leave them and to move on to the next phase of Kara's recovery.

I loved the Pediatric Unit and nurses from the moment we transferred her until Kara was discharged from the hospital July 28. Once again Kara had the room directly across from the nurse's station. She might not have been the sickest patient on the floor, but she needed to be watched closely because of her brain injury. By now, Kara was considered a rehab patient and had a schedule that filled her day with different rehabilitative therapies. The nurses also planned a nursing care schedule which included when they would bathe her, feed her, toilet her and let her nap. They even scheduled her social time.

Kara's dystonic spasms were gone now; they had been replaced with some muscular stiffness and rigidity and tremors but she was much easier to care for than at any other time in her hospital stay. Tom and I kept up our schedule of my being the day parent and his being the evening parent, and I developed a relationship with the day staff as Tom developed the same type of relationship with the evening staff.

Kara's days were busy and so were the nurses, and Tom and I tried to help with Kara's routines as much as we could. It was good for us because it was a safe place for us to learn how to move her from bed to wheelchair and walk her and feed her and perform all of her routine activities of daily living while we had the experts around to critique us and give us suggestions. During the day, I would feed Kara lunch and dinner which were tasks that would take at least a half-hour for each meal. Kara had always been a picky eater and now not only was she still picky, she could only eat foods which were easy to chew so our menu choices for her were extremely limited. She started out by eating only vanilla ice cream in Dixie cups and would eat five or six of those each day until she suddenly stopped. Next she went through her strawberry phase. Then she stopped eating strawberries and moved on to Spaghetti-Os. Just when I thought that perhaps we should buy stock in Chef Boyardee, she stopped eating those and switched to yogurt and applesauce. After I stocked the Pediatric Unit refrigerator with enough yogurt to last a week, she switched to hot dogs and milk shakes. For the last month of her hospital stay, she ate a hot dog for every lunch and dinner. If someone other than me filled out her menu card and neglected to circle the hot dog selection, the kitchen staff would still send up a hot dog on her tray. They knew that Kara was a major hot dog fan, and they were determined not to disappoint her. Maine Medical Center probably set a new record for hot dog consumption for June and July that year.

It was at the end of May while she was a patient on the Pediatric Unit that Kara finally started talking again. Dr. Allan had gone on vacation, and it somehow seemed unjust to me that Kara spoke first to his colleague and not to him, the physician who was so devoted to her and who had had so many interrupted nights of sleep because of her. Dr. Peter Richen was taking care of Dr. Allan's patients that day, and when he came to visit one morning, I said to him casually, "Kara can talk now." Kara was in her wheelchair in the hallway, and he knelt down next to her and said, "What can you say, Kara?" and she said, "Hi" in a deep and throaty whisper. "That is what Walt gets for going on vacation," said Dr. Richen with a grin.

At first it took two people to support Kara as she walked, but gradually she became strong enough that just one person's help was enough. During her free time I would take her for short jaunts up to the playroom or to the television room or to see the little premature babies in the nursery. Her endurance and balance were improving, but every now and then she would loose her balance and end up on the floor. Sometimes she would take me with her.

One night she decided that she was going to get out of bed by herself. At this time Kara was in a fancy Gortex electric air bed with high side rails that was intended to be difficult from which to escape. Carol and Kim, two of the evening nurses, heard strange noises coming from Kara's room. Carol entered the room first to find Kara hanging out of the bed with her head almost touching the floor and her feet straight up in the air. Carol called for Kim to help. They did some complicated gymnastic maneuvers, put Kara right side up and sat her in a chair while they tried to deflate the bed in order to put Kara back into it. The more they tried to deflate the bed, the more the bed inflated, and Kara sat in the chair saying to them, "Bad, bad bed." The nurses got so mad at the "bad, bad bed" that they banished it, and when I arrived the next morning, Kara was in a regular old-fashioned hospital bed. When Dr. Allan told me the story the next morning, I think that he was watching me to see if I might be upset that Kara had decided to take a header off the bed. But she wasn't hurt. I knew that it was an impossible task to watch her every second and as I tried to imagine the scenario of the "bad, bad bed," it seemed as if it could have been a "Saturday Night Live" skit. It became a joke amongst us, and I always admired those nurses for trusting me enough to laugh about that story with me.

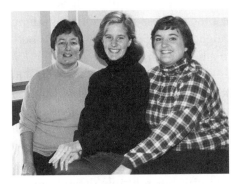

Carol, Kara and Kim on a not-so-bad bed
a year after her discharge.

Tom fell in love with every nurse on the evening shift. One Saturday we were going to a wedding and he was going to meet me at the reception after his "shift" with Kara at the hospital. I asked him if he was going to go home first to get ready. "No," he told me. "I am going to get ready at the hospital and I hope that the nurses are going to bathe me and dress me." I don't think that he was kidding.

The nurses and aides in the Pediatric Unit were an incredible group of people. They amazed me daily with their knowledge, positive attitudes and strength of spirit. Despite the fact that Kara's room was directly across from the nurses' station, I never once heard them discuss another patient; I was always impressed with the confidentiality that they afforded their patients. We never knew another patient's story unless the patient or the parents chose to tell us. Those nurses had a keen sense of when I was sad, and they were right there with open arms and encouraging stories, trying to impart their strength of spirit to me. Since I work in the operating room, all of the parents with whom I deal are anxious and scared as their children go into surgery. I don't need a sixth sense to know that they are sad because they all are. These nurses could discern changes in moods as easily as they could change a diaper. I know that sometimes they must have been sad when one of their patients wasn't doing well or had died, but they never brought that sadness into another patient's room with them. They taught me not only how to be a better nurse but also how to be a better person.

But the biggest privilege of being in the hospital is observing and talking to the parents of the other sick children. There is so much to be learned from them and so much to be shared with them. I met one parent who had a daughter with Down's syndrome who had just had open heart surgery. We were talking in the television room, and she was so proud of her daughter despite her multiple disabilities. She asked me to come in and see her little girl and her attitude made me see not a child with Down's syndrome but a beautiful baby girl with long silky hair on her head that stood straight up and made her look as if she were a little doll. You see, that is the point; she was a little doll who just happened to have Down's syndrome.

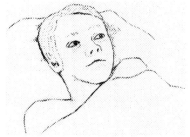

Jesse drawn by his stepfather.

And then there was Jesse, the little boy next door to Kara. He was one of Dr. Allan's patients, too. His condition, torsion dystonia, made him twist and arch uncontrollably as

Kara had done during her worst weeks of dystonia. Dr. Allan introduced Kara to Jesse and would sometimes take Kara into Jesse's room for a visit. They became fond of each other and Jesse often picked out a rose for Kara when he was able to go to the flower shop at Maine Medical Center. As I got to know Jesse and his parents, I began to understand what they were facing as torsion dystonia is a progressive disease. I thought I had achieved a certain level of sophistication but they were way ahead of me in bravery and strength.

There was the little girl who had a big ascitic belly and who was bleeding from her rectum. Just the day before she had been coloring with Kara in the playroom. Now she was being transferred to Boston, so I could only guess how sick she was. I watched the calm resignation on her mother's face; it said "just another setback in a life full of setbacks." There was the mother who was a nurse and she had taken her fifteen-year-old daughter to the emergency room one Sunday for a mononucleosis test and left the emergency room an hour later with a diagnosis of leukemia. It was a totally different illness from Kara's, but just as sudden and just as devastating.

There was also the new mother who had enjoyed a few hours of happiness after her son's birth before learning that he had a serious heart defect requiring immediate surgery. Being twenty-three, she was half my age, but we became friends. She always made me laugh because I never once saw her that she wasn't carrying a big aluminum suitcase that had a breast pump in it. Every time she sat down, she had to pump her breasts. She hated that pump and every day would tell me of her success or failure with it in great detail. Laughter is so therapeutic and every day I looked forward to her stories. I missed her a lot when she went home with her newly healthy little boy. All these parents helped me develop my own approach and attitude toward how I would deal with Kara and her recovery. The most amazing thing was that I never once observed self-pity. These were strong people and I had to emulate them.

So, you can see why I loved this unit. It was a place filled with wonderful people who helped me find acceptance and the courage to maximize every ability that Kara had.

CHAPTER 18

Managed Care?
Somehow we still
manage to care
by Walter Allan, M.D.

⇔ ⇔ ⇔

Once Kara went to the pediatric floor in May the inevitable insurance calls began. When would Kara be able to leave the acute care setting for rehabilitation? The question was a pertinent one. At issue was the hospital bill. Kara's health insurance company wanted to send her to a rehabilitation facility in Brewer, Maine, associated with their company. The facility was three hours from Portland and two and a half hours from Bath where the Anglims lived. Our staff, the Anglims and I wanted Kara to complete her rehabilitation at Maine Medical Center. We were able to justify Kara's stay for awhile on the basis that she had only just had a PEG and ICD placed and, thus, still qualified for "acute" care even though she was nearing her second month in the hospital. However, this would not work for long. We needed to reach a compromise between the cost of a bed at Maine Medical Center and the cost of a bed in the rehabilitation facility in Brewer.

Managed care organizations attempt to control the costs of medical care by auditing how physicians practice. They place certain limitations on what services patients receive and without documentation will not allow these limits to be exceeded. The good companies try to maintain quality at the same time. However, there can be differences of opinion as to what constitutes quality as well as how long services should be rendered. Now, everyone has seen the cartoons about "managed care." For example, there is one that shows an IV bottle with an odometer on it standing next to a befuddled-looking woman in a hospital bed. There is a man in overalls staring at the odometer with a big sign on his back reading "Ajax Managed Care, Limited," with the Limited underlined. The caption reads, "Just here to read the meter, Ma'am." So our view of managed care is a bit befuddled just as the woman in the hospital bed. For physicians, phone calls from managed care nurses are an annoyance on the level of slush on sidewalks, flat tires on the way to work, or a summer cold. But sometimes they are not that bad.

Such was the case with Kara's insurance company, HealthSource. My first call came from a nurse who began by asking politely for an update on Kara rather than opening the conversation with the usual question of when would she be discharged. She obviously knew and understood what Kara and the Anglims were facing. She actually sounded pleased that Kara had been improving. She did get her point in about rehabilitation and their facility in Brewer, but listened when I protested that since Kara was a fourteen-year-old, rehabilitation on the pediatric service of Maine Medical Center might be more appropriate. I added that I thought we had arranged a similar rehabilitation for another young person through a compromise between the hospital and HealthSource. She said she would look into that and would get back to me.

I knew keeping Kara at Maine Medical Center was going to take some effort even if HealthSource was willing to consider it and turned to Carol Zechman, our social worker, to speak to the appropriate hospital administrator. I also spoke to the chief of pediatrics, Dr. Paul Stern, about this plan as he had been interested in setting up a pediatric rehabilitation facility as part of our pediatric service. Carol left numerous voice-mail messages with the administration and Paul had a word with the Vice President of Medical Affairs, Dr. Stephen Larned.

Meanwhile, I heard from one of HealthSource's physicians, Dr. Rob Hochmuth. One of the good things about practicing in one place for two decades is you eventually know everyone in your field. Dr. Hochmuth and I had shared a patient or two over the years and it made it easier for him to listen to my story about Kara. I started as I had done every time I told anyone about Kara—telling how Kara was one of my favorites, about her mother and those yearly Christmas cards she and Kara had sent. Kara's plight was compelling and he understood what we wanted and did not think it was inappropriate for Kara to be rehabilitated at Maine Medical Center, given her age and the family's relationship with us. However, the room rate would have to be a rehab rate. He felt sure that HealthSource would cooperate if the hospital would compromise, but he was not aware that that had ever happened in the past.

Carol Zechman was successful in getting Al Swallow to call me to discuss the issue. He is the hospital's newly appointed vice president for Managed Care. I told him the same story about Kara and added a couple of points about money. Kara had an ICD which alone cost $50,000. I said I was sure her hospitalization was as costly as any pediatric hospitalization I knew of to that point. I added that surely Maine Medical Center and HealthSource could reach a compromise in order to finish the hospital part of her care on the most positive note— and that is exactly what happened.

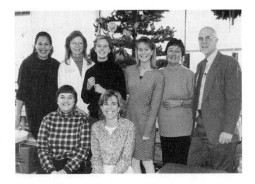

Carol Zechman (third from right, back row) and Kathy Cone (right front row), Kara's hospital tutor, join her and others at Christmas 1996 in the Pediatric Play Room.

But there was more to the money part of Kara's story than the immediate problems of the cost of hospitalization. She was going to need outpatient rehabilitation for a year or more and might need some sort of therapy indefinitely. She would also need to see the cardiologists indefinitely. She would need to have her ICD monitored every few months and its battery changed every few years. At first she would need help in school and at home with tube feedings and medications. Nurses, therapists and doctors were going to be a big expense for an unknown, but prolonged length of time. Eventually the Anglims would run into the cap HealthSource would impose on anyone they insured. This is the sort of thing Carol Zechman knew about. Her first step was to get Kara a Katie Beckett waiver for Medicaid. The ability to qualify for Medicaid without first exhausting all of a family's economic resources is what this waiver allows. How this waiver of Medicaid's usual rules came about is a story worth telling.

Katie Beckett was a six-month-old when she developed a severe viral encephalitis in September 1978 in Cedar Rapids, Iowa. This illness began with a fever and two convulsions. She was hospitalized and her seizures were treated but her condition worsened. She developed paralysis of the muscles of her pharynx and her diaphragm. Because of this she had to be placed on a respirator on the second hospital day. Eventually, her pediatrician, Dr. Tim Ziska, found that Katie had a Coxsackie virus infection. This is one of the viruses that can mimic polio and cause injury to the anterior horn cells in the spinal cord and brainstem.

It was obvious that Katie was intact in other ways as the months passed but she was unable to get off the respirator and unable to leave the hospital. When she was seventeen months of age she was sent to Children's Memorial Hospital in Chicago for a new treatment called a phrenic nerve stimulator. This device which had to be installed surgically had been used in very few children by July 1979. It was supposed to stimulate the nerve to the diaphragm with the hope that Katie could be weaned from her respirator.

However, at the operation it was discovered that her

left phrenic nerve was very atrophic and her right not much better. Back in Cedar Rapids, Katie had the stimulator turned on for increasing lengths of time while she was off respiratory support. At first when the phrenic pacer was tried, her color became dusky and she would sweat after only short periods of time, so she would have to go back on the respirator. Slowly, over the year it was tried, Katie made some strides, being able to stay off the respirator for longer periods. However, as the phrenic pacer did not really seem to be what was helping, it was abandoned. Katie passed her second and third birthdays in the hospital, largely dependent upon the respirator.

But somehow, as time passed, Katie began to make slow improvement. By June 1981 she was able to tolerate long periods of time off the breathing machine when she was awake. That is when her parents began to think of taking Katie home. However, because the Becketts had used up their insurance and Katie would not qualify for federal support out of the hospital, they began to petition the government for help. It made sense to them that Katie would be cared for more cheaply at home. In addition, home would provide a better environment for a developing child. The Becketts' congressman, Tom Tauke, helped them apply for an "exception to policy" for Medicaid coverage of services at home. After frustrating months of review this "exception" was rejected. This prompted Congressman Tauke to approach Vice President George Bush with the details of Katie's case. Vice President Bush approached President Reagan and he granted the exception. On December 19, 1981, at age three years, eight months Katie Beckett went home.

Katie's mother felt the exception Katie got should be extended to other children with similar needs. Congress eventually saw the wisdom of this and the Katie Beckett waiver was created. Interestingly, Katie Beckett has grown up and is an honor student at her Cedar Rapids high school. During the recent public forums on health care convened by Hillary Clinton in President Clinton's first term, Katie testified about her medical needs and those of people like her. Katie still has a tracheostomy and when she gets viral illnesses needs to go back on a respirator for several days. So Katie at age seventeen still needs the Katie Beckett waiver. As there was no way of predicting how Kara would do over a lifetime, the Katie Beckett waiver was a very helpful addition to the Anglims' insurance coverage.

CHAPTER 19

Parsimonious

෯ ෯ ෯

Kara was in the hospital from April 7 until July 28 and during those four months Maine Medical Center was her home, and the staff was her temporary extended family. Maine Medical Center became a huge part of Tom's and my lives, too—both medically and socially. We saw and talked more to hospital personnel and patients' families than any of our other friends. And amidst all of the pathos of hospital life we found hope, humor or at least amusement with every experience. The varied personalities constantly intrigued Tom and me. Most of these experiences were positive except for Kara and my interaction with one team member. You can't like everybody and everybody can't like you.

While Kara was a patient on the Pediatric Unit, we had regular team meetings regarding her progress. At these conferences, each specialty team dealing with Kara had a representative present who would give a brief overview of Kara's progress and their goal for the next step in her rehabilitation. The members would be able to ask questions of each other and offer suggestions, and Tom and I had the opportunity to voice any concerns or questions that we had. These meetings were usually attended by Dr. Allan, the physiatrist, nurses, physical therapists, occupational therapists, speech therapists, the neuropsychologist, the social worker, the nutritionist, the resident-of-the-month and any other interested specialists. These meetings took about an hour and were informative sessions that helped Tom and me understand Kara's prognosis and helped all of us plan for her future. These meetings were always objective and realistic assessments of Kara's returning skills, and yet it was hard for most of the team members not to be optimistic as we watched Kara's cognitive and motor skills slowly but steadily improve. It was easy to assess the members' personalities as they spoke; they wore their hearts on their sleeves.

But then there was one other person at the team meeting. I don't need to describe this person; all that you need to know is that this member of the team was the reincarnation of Eeyore from *Winnie the Pooh*. As you might recall, Eeyore was the character who was always negative. If someone said, "Oh, what a beautiful day. The sky is blue," Eeyore would say, "Oh, but I see a cloud." It was the same with this person.

At the first team meeting, Eeyore was the last to speak after listening to all of the other specialists summarize their assessments of Kara's progress. Eeyore expressed shock that the other members of the team could see so much potential for Kara's recovery while Eeyore could see none. "We have to be parsimonious with our diagnosis," Eeyore proclaimed, "and blah, blah, blah," on and on. I had no idea what the word "parsimonious" meant, but I knew that in this context, it definitely had a negative connotation. I decided I was not going to listen to another word that Eeyore said, and I spent the rest of the time trying to figure out what the word "parsimonious" meant and why Eeyore had the need to use a word of which few people in the room probably knew the definition. This was my defense mechanism against a message I didn't want to hear. "It is definitely an SAT word," I thought, having had a daughter who had just taken that test twice. "It sort of reminds me of a parsnip or persimmon," I thought, but I knew that didn't fit into the meaning of the sentence. I whispered to Tom, "What does "parsimonious" mean?" He shrugged his shoulders. I made a mental note that the next time I would bring a dictionary to one of these meetings. Then I remembered that Tom had told me in one of his evening conversations with Dr. Allan that the topic had come up that Dr. Allan would have liked to have become an English professor if he hadn't become a physician. I also knew that he read a lot so I thought that maybe he would know what the definition of "parsimonious" was.

After the meeting Dr. Allan had wanted to show us

Kara's MRI and had it up on the X-ray view box in the conference room so that he could discuss it with us. But first things had to come first. "Dr. Allan, what does parsimonious mean?" He did know and he told me that it meant stingy or miserly. "Well, then Eeyore used it incorrectly because the words parsimonious and diagnosis don't go together," I insisted. "Well," said Dr. Allan, "actually there is such a thing as a parsimonious diagnosis. What Eeyore wanted to say was that in Eeyore's experience the team was being overly optimistic and that didactic proof for such optimism was lacking." "Well, then Eeyore isn't looking," I said, "and I am not going to listen to that." Dr. Allan had told me that he would tell me if and when to stop being optimistic, and he hadn't told me to stop yet and until he did, I was not going to listen to the possibility of a parsimonious diagnosis.

So "parsimonious" became a joke between our family and Dr. Allan. It must have been Eeyore's word-of-the-week because Eeyore used it often for the next week and then never said it again, much to our chagrin. But that was the beginning of nothing but trouble between Eeyore and me. We never did agree on anything and Eeyore was the cause of the only time that I swore in Kara's entire hospital stay. One day Eeyore told me that it was time to start doing psychotherapy with Kara. I don't know much about psychotherapy, but I do know that it entails being able to have a dialogue between the therapist and the client. At the point that Eeyore wanted to start this, Kara was capable of only the simplest communication, and I felt that the thought of psychotherapy was totally off-base at this stage of Kara's recovery. She could basically only say "yes" or "no" and even those answers were not always accurate. But Dr. Allan was on vacation and I couldn't ask him what was right; Tom was at work so I couldn't ask him his opinion; I knew that I had to take charge. "She can't fucking talk. How do you think that you are going to do psychotherapy with her? You are not to do anything with her until Dr. Allan comes back from vacation and he can be part of this decision." I felt like Nancy Reagan: JUST SAY NO!

Actually, I am grateful for meeting Eeyore and having

to deal with all this. Eeyore taught me a lot. I learned how to avoid unpleasant visits from people. Kara and I would pretend that we were asleep when we saw Eeyore walk onto the nursing unit. It was an effective method of avoidance and it saved me plenty of aggravation. I learned that no matter how smart someone is, sometimes a mother is smarter. I learned that it is possible to stop a process that doesn't seem appropriate until I could get input from people that I trusted. And finally I learned that there was no need for a parsimonious diagnosis for Kara as we watched her get better and planned for her return to our home.

CHAPTER 20

Eleanor Roosevelt and Me

తుతుత

The point of Kara being in the hospital was for her to recover to the point where cardiologically and rehabilitatively she was well enough to return home. Our home was empty without her and we knew that her being home with us was the best rehabilitative medicine available but it was a change that was loaded with emotional and medical and logistical issues. Even though I was so happy that Kara could come home instead of having to go to a residential rehabilitation facility, her journey home was a difficult time for me.

First of all, Kara and I were leaving the protective confines of the hospital. Even though Tom and I were with Kara a lot, the nursing staff and therapists delivered a good percentage of Kara's physical care each day. They took care of her each night, and Tom and I could sleep knowing that she was well cared for in our absence. Each morning the nurses bathed her so that when I arrived at the hospital she was all clean, dressed in her tee shirt and shorts and had a new hair style. They fed her breakfast, sang along with her tapes and lovingly talked with her. Now it would all be up to Tom and me. The physical care which we had to provide for Kara at this point was extensive. She could walk, but only if someone took her arm and supported her greatly, and then only for about 200 feet. She could sit in a chair, but only if someone helped her into it and out of it. She could drink from a glass, but only if there were a straw in it and someone guided it into her mouth. She could use the toilet, but only if we undid her pants and helped her onto the toilet. She could eat, but only if someone put each spoonful in her mouth. She could enjoy our company and follow our conversations, but she could not entertain herself.

But there was more than just her physical care that I was going to miss. With Kara's room being right across from the nurses' station, I only had to poke my head out the door to have instant company and conversation. It resembled living in a college dormitory where there was always someone available with whom to have fun. Those nurses were smart because about two weeks before Kara's discharge date, Kara was moved to a room down the hall. I came to the hospital one day to find a stranger in Kara's room. Someone was sicker than Kara and needed the special attention that was afforded the patient in that room. "So," I joked, "the next move is out the door." It wasn't really a joke because I knew it was true. Our hospital neighbors asked us, "Did you move to a more up-scale area?" and I would answer, "Yes, we didn't like our old neighbors." I was hopelessly addicted to the routine and personality of Maine Medical Center and by moving a little closer to the door, I was being gently weaned from what had become my little world. I needed to develop new routines for our family, and I had to reinvent a new world where Tom and I were the primary caregivers for our daughter. I was not going to have instantly available emotional support and I knew that I was going to have to rely much more upon my own inner strength. I was scared because I wasn't really sure that I could do this.

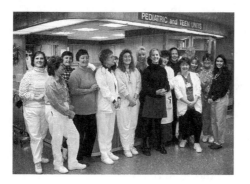

Nurses, therapists and doctors with Kara on the pediatric ward at Christmas 1996.

There were even more issues than this for me. On the Pediatric Unit at Maine Medical Center, most of the children are very sick. I don't think that I ever met one child there who was merely having his tonsils out or his hernia repaired. This was not a hospital for the routine pediatric problems. This was a hospital where many of the patients were having chemotherapy for various cancers or leukemia, and these bald patients bravely wheeled their IVs up and down the halls. This was a hospital where children were recovering from traumatic brain injuries as their parents encouraged their rehabilitation. This was a hospital where children with serious heart problems were being treated. The parents of these children pushed them around the ward in their wheelchairs or wagons accompanied by oxygen tanks and tubings. Not many of the patients looked healthy and they shouldn't, after all they were in the hospital.

But now we were going home. In the hospital, it was easier to accept Kara's handicaps because that was the reason that she was in the hospital, but at home, she should be healthy. She was supposed to bounce down the steps telling me, "Mom, Kate and I are going to ride our bikes to Vanessa's house." In my heart, I wanted her to come back the way that she left the morning of April 7th. However, that wasn't our reality and as wonderful as it was that she was coming home, it was hard to see her come home so differently from the way she left that Friday morning, walking down the street with her blue L.L. Bean backpack, blithely meeting her friends for their walk to the bus stop. My heart was breaking, but I knew that I couldn't let it show; if I showed anything less than courage and humor and perseverance and optimism, I wouldn't be doing my best for Kara and our family. Her recovery hinged upon Tom and Guerin and me, and we could not ever let her down.

I once saw a show on Eleanor Roosevelt who had the philosophy of not ever letting anyone see her cry. When she was sad, she would go in the bathroom and run the water loudly and cry her eyes out. I can't tell you how many times I did this. I would take a bath and let the water and the tears flow. Our water bill must have decreased during this time because the tub was always half-filled with tears.

It was true that my life had been turned upside down in a heartbeat, and I suppose that I had reason to feel angry or bitter or jealous of people with "normal" lives. But as I analyzed my feelings, I would come to the conclusion that it wasn't really me who had my life turned upside down, it was Kara's life that was altered in every way. I could still tie my shoes; she could not. I could feed myself; she could not. I could walk where I wanted; she could not. I could communicate every need; she could not. And then I would look at her sweet little face that showed that she was capable of only the most innocent thoughts. I would think of her determination to regain her independence. I would look into her eyes and see the purest form of trust. It was obvious what my course of action had to be. I couldn't dwell on the negative. I had to be able to look upon this phase of our lives in twenty years and smile and say, "Yes, I did my best."

The main controversy that surrounded Kara's discharge was the question to which facility she should be discharged. She was mobile and could walk with help, but she needed assistance with every activity of daily living, from eating to bathing to toiletting. She needed a high level of rehabilitative services which would include occupational, speech and physical therapy. She was a candidate for a residential rehabilitative facility, but there is no place in the state of Maine that serves the residential pediatric rehabilitative needs. The facilities that do exist in the state were willing to bend their age rules to accept Kara into their facility, but Tom and I thought that we could provide Kara's daily care if she could be accepted into an outpatient rehabilitative facility from which she could come home each evening. She was a patient who fell between the cracks because she was not really handicapped enough for residential rehab, but she was a little too handicapped for outpatient rehab. Fortuitously, there exists in Portland an outpatient rehabilitation facility called BaySide. They interviewed Kara, Tom and me, listened and observed and then decided to accept Kara into their program. I hoped the combination of BaySide's skill and Kara's life at home filled with friends and family would make her progress continuous and her attitude upbeat. The time of indecision while we were contemplating the pros and cons of outpatient versus inpatient rehabilitation was difficult because Tom and I wanted to make the correct decision. We tried to be carefully logical and objective but in the end, our hearts ruled. We wanted Kara home with us.

Friday, July 28th was chosen for Kara's discharge date and the thought of her discharge created a dichotomy of attitudes for me. I was happy because the sick little girl we had brought to the hospital in a coma four months ago was now going home with ever-returning abilities. I was sad because these were the people who had saved her life, and I was attached to them, and now I was leaving them. I was scared because I had no idea of what this new life would be like for our family, or if I could handle it, or if I would fail. I was exhausted because the planning of Kara's return home required my retelling and reliving her story to every new person involved in her care. Everyone kept saying to me, "You must be so glad to have Kara coming home." I answered, "Yes," to everyone, but anyone who knew me well must have known that it was only a half-hearted "yes." There were so many emotions involved in the move home, and happiness was only one of them.

But I knew that we had to imitate the Nike commercial and "Just do it" and that is what we did. We had to put aside our fears and worries and approach Kara's homecoming with the same vigor and commitment and optimism with which we approached every other phase of her illness. I dreaded the day we left the hospital because I am the worst saying-good-bye-person in the world. I am fine until someone says something nice to me, and then the tears just start and don't easily stop. I kept saying to the people who had become our friends over those four months, "I'm fine. Just don't say anything nice to me." It took me until about noon to say good-bye to everyone and then we left the protective custody of Maine Medical Center to start this next phase of Kara's recovery.

We had changed the living room into Kara's bedroom complete with hospital bed and pump for her feeding tube. We had made the downstairs bathroom hers. I had taken two weeks off from work to develop a routine, and my parents were there to help with the housework and cooking while I took care of Kara. Transitions are not easy for me but this one actually went smoothly. It helped a great deal that I am a nurse; I didn't need to learn any new skills; I only had to adapt what skills I had to fit Kara's needs.

Somehow I made it through, but I can assure you that this, for me, was definitely the most difficult phase of Kara's recovery. What was hard was seeing the pity in people's eyes when they saw Kara for the first time, hearing the doubt of Kara's recovery in their voices, and not knowing if this was going to be my life for a day or forever. But even though the loss was sudden and the recovery slow, the lesson to be learned was that with the help and love of family and friends as well as her own healing process, Kara could and would recover. Even though our lives had been tragically altered once, I trusted in the belief that they could be altered again, but this time with a happy ending. I believe that fairy tales can come true.

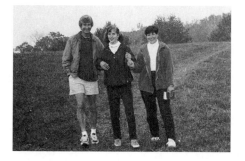

*Tom, Kara and Maryann on a walk
after three months out of the hospital.*

৵৵৵

PART II

LESSONS

CHAPTER 21

Lobbying

ↄ ↄ ↄ

Kara came home on a Friday and started going to BaySide Rehabilitation on Monday. This facility was interested in Kara because she presented many new challenges to them, and they were looking forward to working with her and hoping to make a significant impact on her recovery. Most of their patients were brain-injured as the result of trauma so Kara's hypoxic brain injury was something different for them. I have learned that there are both similarities and differences in the recovery phase of these two types of injuries, and BaySide was enthusiastically embracing the prospect of all the new knowledge they would attain from helping Kara. BaySide is a little community within a community, and I am constantly amazed at the professional but friendly balance they maintain with their clients.

BaySide was wonderful with Kara. They used all of her interests to facilitate her recovery and were clever and innovative with their program. They knew that Kara's favorite candy was Skittles and Skittles just happened to be one of the candies in their vending machine. They incorporated this interest into Kara's rehabilitative plan. If Kara wanted Skittles, she had to walk to the machine, put her money in, press the appropriate buttons and then open the candy bag and use her own hands to feed herself. As most teenagers, Kara loves the radio and music and so much of Kara's therapy was done to the beat of her favorite tunes. Kara also enjoys shopping and so BaySide would have Kara walk to the local stores, buy small items, and be accountable for the financial transactions.

One of their main goals for Kara was for her to return to public high school in Bath. As wonderful as BaySide was, all of their clients were older than Kara and they could not meet all of her social needs and academic needs. So with BaySide and Dr. Allan as our allies, Tom and I ventured into our first meeting with the Bath School Department as we progressed towards getting Kara back into school. It was intimidating for me because I didn't know many of the school officials at this meeting. These same officials had a limited understanding of Kara's condition, and yet they were the ones upon whom the success or failure of this next phase of Kara's recovery depended.

What I found is that the school department did not listen to Tom and me, but they sure did listen to Dr. Allan and the rehabilitative specialists. I call them my "lobby group" and I know that Kara would not be having as successful a school year without their input. For example, when Kara first reentered the school, the school wanted her to be transported from class to class in a wheelchair. She had been walking with assistance for months when this wheelchair idea was thrust upon us and I was aghast. "How can you possibly think that putting her in a wheelchair is a good idea? It is setting back her rehab, making Kara even more different than her peers, and it is unnecessary. She will have an aide with her constantly and that is all she needs." We were engaged in verbal fisticuffs. I had to ask both BaySide and Dr. Allan to call or write a letter to the school department stating the unnecessary nature of the wheelchair before the school would consent to allowing Kara to walk to her classes. BaySide's strength is not only in their rehabilitative abilities but also in their role as fierce advocates for their handicapped clients. Nothing gets in the way of their advocacy and I have used them often in this role.

In fairness to Kara's school system, BaySide has told me that they have never been involved with a system that has been so cooperative and willing to adapt to a client's needs. Even though at times this has taken some work, in the long run, Kara's needs have been well met with flexibility and she has been surrounded with teachers who are both skilled and compassionate.

So after much planning, many meetings and a fair

amount of anguish, Kara was all set to return to school two days per week in October. Once again the word "bittersweet" comes to my mind as I describe what it was like for me. First of all, her gait was too unsteady for her to take the school bus as all of the other neighborhood children do. So after years of her running down the hill to hop on the bus at the last possible moment, our friend Margie, who was a high school senior at the time, stopped by our house every Tuesday and Thursday morning. Then Tom or I drove them to school where Margie took Kara's arm and escorted her through the crowds of kids gathered outside the school and delivered her to her aide, Janice. I would drive off quickly after I dropped them at school because if I stopped to consider what a sad picture they presented, I would start every day with tears—Margie, tall and straight and protective; Kara, a wounded little bird. Picking Kara up at school was just as difficult for me, but I learned a little avoidance mechanism. I learned to pick Kara up after all of the other kids had left, and then the contrast between their bouncy steps and her halting ones didn't have to be as obvious. There was a time when we were not sure that Kara was going to survive and if she did that she would have a meaningful recovery and now, here she was back at school. So, of course I was happy. But yet I wasn't happy because she wasn't taking English and History and Algebra as her classmates were; she was taking occupational therapy and physical therapy and speech therapy. But I cannot allow myself to look at what isn't there for Kara; I have to look at what is there and be happy for what skills return every day. Someday I will probably have a gigantic ulcer from having such opposing emotions.

I can't help but carry the sad part in my heart, and I am lucky that I have a few special people who help me with that part of Kara's recovery. They never have said to me, "Maryann, you are boring and we are tired of talking about your emotions." They always listen and help and I listen to them, too. They are the ones who make it possible for me to be hopelessly optimistic, to look beyond today and to make the transition from a hospital mom to a regular mom.

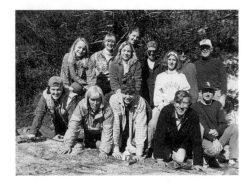

Fall family hike with Kara including the Coes, Van Ordens, Allans and Anglims.

CHAPTER 22

Guerin

లాలాలా

When Kara became ill, Guerin was in the final weeks of her senior year at Morse High School. This was supposed to be an exciting and carefree time of her life. She had been accepted at Providence College, academic expectations were all but over at her high school, the senior prom was just around the corner, the weather was warming and the beach was beckoning. But the phone call that she received while she was swimming in Florida changed all that. Her life of limited responsibilities and her role in the family all had to be reassessed and new patterns had to develop quickly and effectively in order for Tom and me to do our best for Kara, Guerin and each other.

Guerin was at the stage of her life where she was developing her independence from Tom and me and was closely tied to her friends, many of whom she had known since kindergarten. She never complained about the many hours that Tom and I devoted to Kara. I think she tolerated our preoccupation with Kara because it kept us from interfering in her life. Guerin has been involved in her share of mischievous events and I am sure that Tom and I only know about half of them, but she is a good and responsible daughter who knows right from wrong.

Most of the parents of Guerin's friends were our friends, too, and that was a big source of consolation for us. Every night that I stayed at the hospital later than I should have, Guerin always had a home and good meal at the house of one of those friends. She never lacked for love or attention because if her own parents couldn't provide it that day, one of her "surrogate parents" could. They also made sure that Guerin got down to Portland to see Kara at the hospital whenever she wanted.

It was difficult for Guerin to find the right balance between her responsibilities. She needed to spend ample time studying to keep her grades acceptable for Providence College; she needed to enjoy her friends so that she wouldn't resent time spent with Kara; she needed to fulfill her obligation as a sister helping Kara with her recovery; she needed to help with some household chores that Tom and I no longer had time for, and she needed to be safe and assure us that all of her social decisions were mature ones so that we could be free of the usual parents-of-teenagers' worries. She had to be able to look to the future but know that when she looked back on this time of her life she had tried her best to be fair to herself, to Kara and to us.

Tom and I knew what a difficult balancing act this was going to be as we struggled with some of the same dilemmas. We knew that Guerin needed autonomy and had the right to make many of her own decisions but we also knew how dangerous the end of senior year is for these young adults of the nineties. We desperately needed her to be safe. We already had one daughter in the hospital with a brain injury, and we didn't want anything to happen to Guerin. Tom did a better job of finding the correct balance than I did; he could trust her judgment, whereas I had to know where she was, how she was getting there and whom she was with at any given moment. We knew that Guerin could physically take care of herself, but certainly she needed us for emotional support, and we had to be sure to save enough of ourselves to give it to her.

One evening I came home from the hospital to find Guerin in tears over her schoolbooks. She was still catching up on her schoolwork from her week in Florida and was feeling overwhelmed with homework and the seriousness of Kara's condition. I held her in my arms and rocked her, just as if she were eight instead of eighteen. We had two daughters, both needy in their own way, and we had the awesome responsibility of taking care of them both. Helping Guerin cope with Kara's illness was just as important as guiding Kara back to good health.

Guerin did find her niche in Kara's recovery process.

It was helping with Kara's biweekly water therapy along with the recreational therapist in the pool at the Portland YMCA. It was a job that took a good part of Guerin's day and it was an important part of Kara's rehabilitation. Every Monday and Wednesday during June and July, Guerin would drive to Portland to be a part of this therapy. It involved getting Kara changed into her bathing suit, transferring Kara into her wheelchair and then into the van, driving to the YMCA and getting her into the pool area, an hour of water therapy and then reversing the process to get Kara back to the hospital. This routine took about five hours each day and Guerin unfailingly completed it every week. She also learned how to deliver every aspect of Kara's physical care, including the tube feedings, and could efficiently and patiently perform these nursing skills as well as Tom or I. Guerin would make a great nurse, doctor, or rehabilitation therapist, but she is interested in Spanish and wants to live in Spain and has no interest in the health sciences.

Now as I write this, Guerin is a sophomore in college. I know that Kara misses her and I know that Guerin feels guilty about not being closer to home and Kara during this recovery phase. But just as Tom and I had to return to our jobs and our lives apart from Kara, so did Guerin. College is where she should be. When she comes home, she proudly takes Kara shopping or to the show or to McDonald's and thinks that Kara is the most amazing and bravest sister in the whole world.

Guerin now has a maturity and intangible attitude which only come from surviving a rough experience in a positive way. She is devoted to her sister and treats her with gentle love and humor. She has been able to find the correct balance of self and selflessness and she has been one of the most important contributors to Kara's recovery. She has seen and lived a part of life that most nineteen-year-olds haven't and has integrated these experiences sweetly into her personality. For a parent, these are some of the bittersweet dividends of Kara's story.

CHAPTER 23

Thomas

෬ ෬ ෬

Usually I call my husband "Tom" except when I want him to pay attention to me and then he becomes "Thomas." He is the person who always makes me laugh, and I am the person who keeps his life interesting. If it weren't for me, he would have no stories to tell his patients as they sit in his dental chair. I am the person with the imagination to find adventure in the most mundane events and he is my audience. I am the compulsive person who wants everything to be done my way and immediately. He is the gentle person who doesn't care if I had time to cook dinner or not. He is the smarter of us, but I have all the common sense. I am the person who artistically decides how the outside of the house will be decorated for Christmas, and he is the person who climbs up on the ladder in the freezing cold to string the lights. I am the spoiled brat who says, "The grass is too long," and he is the mature person who cuts it. I am the organized one who plans everything; Tom is the thinker. I am fast about getting things done and I never procrastinate while Tom is meticulous and slow to get started. I make everything fun but Tom is the patient one. I am the loud, talkative one and Tom is the quiet listener. I can be quick-tempered while he is reasonable. I quickly assess any problem and, right or wrong, have an immediate plan while he is still trying to determine the nature of the problem and develop a philosophy of problem solving.

We have totally opposite strengths and weaknesses, and I have come to believe that this was a good thing for Kara. If we were both like me, we would have known the exact number of calories that Kara needed, but neither one of us would have had a calm enough demeanor to feed her patiently. If we were both like Tom, she would be slowly fed morsel by morsel and not have any time for speech or occupational or physical therapy. The differences in our personalities became an asset for Kara's recovery and I think that our two styles combined to form one effective style.

The differences in our personalities were only too obvious to the Special Care Unit nurses. They are used to not only helping the critically ill patients in their care, but also offering the emotional support that is so important to the families. I was able to talk easily to them, and I was able to let them see me cry, maybe because we were all women and moms and nurses. They could help me because they knew my emotional state either intuitively or because I was busily telling them.

Tom was a different story. One day, one of the nurses said to me, "How is your husband doing? We really worry about the quiet ones." I do think the quiet ones have a harder time; I externalized most of my anxieties while Tom internalized them. You could tell just by looking at him. When Kara collapsed April 7, Tom had a full beard. That plus the worry and sadness on his face made him look ten years older overnight. Finally Linda told him that he had to shave his beard and then he only looked five years older.

You cannot make someone talk who doesn't want to, but I usually could get to understand some of his feelings by asking him questions. "What did you think when you got the phone call from the hospital? How fast did you drive down to Maine Medical Center? What did you think while you were driving? Did you know what happened to Kara while you were driving? Did you listen to the radio while you were driving or did you just worry? Did you know that Linda and I were with her in the ambulance? How much do you love me and do you think that we will survive this?" I have learned not to wait for Tom to tell me his feelings; I just ask him. He hates these questions and has a tolerance for about five and then that is it until another day.

I knew from various life experiences that tragic events can often dissolve a marriage. I knew it from my friend Terry who had delivered a stillborn baby about fifteen years ago.

She and her husband had gone to a support group called Empty Arms and of the five or six couples involved in the group, only she and her husband were still married. I knew that Guerin and Kara needed an intact family to make it through this turbulent time and that Tom and I needed to work hard, not only to help Kara regain her health, but to keep our marriage strong.

We had our twenty-third wedding anniversary while Kara was in the hospital and on that day I was contemplating our wedding vows. Tom and I promised to marry "for better or for worse, for richer or poorer, in sickness and in health, 'til death do us part." In Catholic school, we learned that a vow is a solemn promise and I believe that. The resolve of our wedding vows was definitely being tested because we were seeing the "worse" and the "poorer" and the "sickness" but we had promised each other to stand by each other through anything and a promise is a promise.

This should be the stage of our lives when Tom and I should be finding time for our own leisure activities and travel together, but due to Kara's illness we are forced to devote most of our leisure activities and time to her. It is easy to enjoy being with Kara; she is sweet, funny, hard-working and committed to her recovery and she will try to do anything that you ask her. It is an honor to be part of her life and it is fascinating to watch her skills return. But still this is not how we would have planned our lives.

One day I told Tom that I thought that there were a lot of forty-seven-year-old men who would look at a situation such as ours and leave it, saying that they wanted to have their lives back. He said that I was wrong and that "no man would desert his child," but I don't think so. When I see Tom's devotion to Kara and the level of physical and emotional care that he provides her, I know that he believes in our wedding vows, too.

On a day-to-day basis, it is the little irritating habits that will make the opposite spouse crazy. So I try extra hard to leave the bath mat over the side of the tub and not on the floor and I try hard not to leave the garage door open after I drive the car into the garage; Tom tries not to leave twelve pairs of shoes by the kitchen door and tries hard to remember to carry the laundry basket upstairs when it is sitting at the bottom of the steps. We know that we are sailing in treacherous waters, but we are using all of our skills to stay safe.

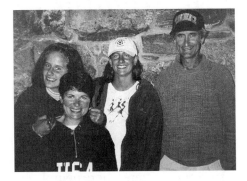

The tannest Anglims in Maine, summer 1996.

CHAPTER 24

Et in Arcadia Ego
by Walter Allan, M.D.

ی ی ی

By July Kara had made significant strides and was getting ready to go home. She had gone from coma through the restless, severely dystonic state where neurologic progress was difficult. When that finally stopped in June she began to make very slow strides with the help of her nurses, therapists and her family. Her neurologic status in July was much better but she still required a lot of assistance. She needed a wheelchair to go any long distance and her gait was very stiff and slow with a short stride. She needed help with eating, washing herself and toiletting because of her dystonic hand and arm muscles. Her speech was coming along but she was still very difficult to understand, and often would start any reply to a question by repeating whatever was said to her. Kara now faced months more of working to return as close as possible to what she was like before her cardiac arrest.

A good rule-of-thumb for neurologic recovery is to say that it can continue for at least a year in adults and perhaps as long as two years in kids. But this is a gross oversimplification and no one knows for sure how long cognitive recovery can continue. Why it is that things can continue to improve for that long a period, or longer, is not known but must have to do with the self-organizing powers of the brain and its systems. After all, that is what the brain is all about: self-organizing systems designed to adapt to the myriad of internal and external signals it processes each millisecond. Out of all that processing, our movements, thoughts and personalities emerge. And, of course, we still do not have much more than half-worked out theories about how these things "emerge" from all

116

those cells doing their jobs. The question "How do thoughts arise?" is part of what is called the mind/body problem. This question has been debated by philosophers for centuries with little progress even in our own enlightened time of PET scans, MRI scans and computers. The good news for Kara was that we do not have to know how it works for progress to occur in her recovery. This was a matter more for her and her family than it was for any specific treatment. Kara's own personality and doggedness with her family's support was what was most likely to get her better. Her therapists and the rehabilitation doctors were there to be the guides.

My job for much of Kara's hospitalization was to interpret for her family, the nurses and therapists why one thing or another was happening on Kara's road to recovery. Since I usually did not know, I would fall back on quasi-philosophical explanations like the one above about self-organizing systems. And now and then I might bring up the mind/body problem. This became a joke with the Anglims. Especially when I let it drop one evening that I had to leave a conversation we were having to go to my mind/body problem discussion group. They grinned as they asked what we might be discussing at such a group. When it came out that our recent readings were articles entitled, "What It's Like to Be a Bat" and "The Beliefs and Desires of a Thermostat," my fate with the Anglims was sealed. I am sure they thought of me as kindly, but now I was also thought of as crazy or at least eccentric. Kindly, crazy and eccentric, Dr. Allan. Since I thought of myself that way, maybe it was not so bad. In any event, it was through these sorts of moments that we began to become more than just professionally attached. We began to become friends.

I had to work very hard to maintain some professional distance from Kara and her parents. They were often, if not always, the subject of dinner conversation between my wife and me during those three-and-a-half months. This was partly because of Kara's compelling story but partly because of who they are. Everyone likes the Anglims. It also had to do with the amount of time I spent with them. I saw Kara twice a day and often spent an hour in the evening talking about all manner of things with her parents. A lot of these chats would be about what they or Guerin were doing away from the hospital. But eventually the pressing questions I could never really answer would come out. Questions about how Kara felt as she went through the severe dystonic spasms. Or what it meant when Kara cried. Or could I see any recent progress. Maryann was more likely to ask these questions than Tom. But that was how their relationship worked. The good thing was they were both able to accept that I did not know the answers.

To maintain some distance, I consistently called Tom and Maryann "Dr. Anglim" and "Mrs. Anglim" throughout Kara's hospitalization. One evening I had finished my visit with Kara and Tom and was on my way out of the hospital when I recalled something I needed to tell Tom. So I called the pediatric nurses' station and asked them to get him to the phone. He answered and I said, "Doc, I forgot to tell you..." and he interrupted me in midsentence. "You must have the wrong person. This is Tom Anglim." After a little embarrassment over being so formal, I told him what I wanted to say. For quite a while thereafter he always called me "Doc" and I reciprocated. This was Tom's style. During his evening "Kara duty" he would entertain Kara, the nurses and me with his latest jokes. These were usually puns of the worst variety, the type he always had to tell a second time before any of us would get it. Except perhaps Kara, who had heard them all before. Without much prompting we could usually get her to say, "Dumb!" in answer to the question, "What do you think of Dad's joke, Kara?" I think Tom's favorite joke was the following:

Tom: "What did the termite say when he walked into the bar?
Listener: "I don't know."
Tom: "Is the bartender here?"
Listener: "Ah, what?"
Tom: "Is the bar TENDER here?"
Listener: "Groan!"

Maryann was just as funny but without jokes. Her humor usually turned on herself, Tom or her friends. I felt I was becoming a friend as I became included in her jokes. I have season tickets to Portland's double-A baseball team, the Sea Dogs. Once Maryann found out I was a Sea Dog fan she paid close attention to their schedule and the outcome of the games. I would give away my tickets to friends when I could not go to a game. It rains a lot in Portland in the spring and often when I gave away the tickets the Sea Dogs would have a rain-out. Maryann accused me of knowing this was going to happen before giving away the tickets. "Oh, I see it was another Sea Dog rain-out last night. I bet Dr. Allan gave somebody his tickets, Kara," she would say when she would see me on morning rounds. Then she would take it a step further, "Have you ever given your tickets away on a nice day, Dr. Allan?" But by then I knew her sense of humor and answered, "Not knowingly."

I was able to keep up my professional facade until Kara was discharged. But I gave it up when the Van Ordens invited my wife, Ann, and I to sail with them, the Anglims and the Coes. These two families had been unwavering in their support of the Anglims. Just as I found the daily visits by both Tom and Maryann to be exceptional in my experience, so I found the daily, ongoing, long-term support these two families provided the Anglims to be unusual.

Linda would come to see Kara in Maryann's place when Maryann had to be at work. She often accompanied Maryann when Tom could not get away from his dental practice and something important or stressful was occurring in Kara's care. Linda, her daughters, Emily and Julia, and her husband, Rufus often visited on weekends. These visits were especially exciting for Kara as the daughters are Kara's long-term friends. Linda's oldest daughter, Michelle, lived in Portland after graduating from college that spring.

And she, too, could be counted on to spend time with Kara if Maryann or Linda could not make the day shift. Michelle saw Kara almost daily at one point in Kara's course and became very interested in how the speech, occupational and physical therapists handled Kara despite all of her problems. It became a life-changing experience for Michelle. She got a job at Maine Medical Center as an occupational therapy aide and plans to get her degree in occupational therapy.

John Van Orden is an orthopedic surgeon who has known Maryann since she first took a job as an operating room nurse at Midcoast Hospital. Their families were close and John and his daughters, Barbara and Margie, had known Kara and Guerin since they were toddlers. John included the girls in many of his leisure activities—from sailing and kayaking, to camping and hiking. Kara was one of his crew during the sailboat racing season. So John thought it would be good for Kara to go sailing again. I did not believe he could pull this off, given how unsteady Kara was, but he did and by all accounts Kara loved it. His daughters were very attached to Kara, especially Margie who was a high school junior. She was a runner and a swimmer just like Kara and Guerin and was at the top of her form that spring.

The first time Kara left the hospital in early June she went to the regional championship track meet to see Guerin and Margie run. Margie was favored to win the mile that day but it did not happen. She fainted in the middle of the event. This had never happened before, but because Kara's story was on everyone's mind, it precipitated a cardiac workup. The diagnosis was supraventricular ectopic pacemaker that was successfully ablated by Joel Cutler. John Van Orden calls Kara "Margie's angel" and thanks to the close relationship these families share, they got through Margie's ordeal easily.

So Ann and I knew it was something to be invited for a Labor Day sail and a meal with these three families at the Van Ordens' house. I knew John from mutual patients over the years, and I knew his wife Joanna because she had been a special education teacher who taught some of the children I saw in my office. But we were still surprised by the invitation. It signaled a change in my relationship with all of these people. The first thing I said when I saw the Anglims at this party was we were going to have to call each other by our first names. By this time I no longer had any professional distance from them in my heart of hearts anyway.

It was a beautiful day. John lives on the New Meadows

River in a picturesque setting called Shoal Cove. He has a gaff-rigged catboat that could take all eight adults. He borrowed a friend's catboat to accommodate the kids. When we got to their house it was nearly low tide which meant a steep descent down to their dock where the two catboats were rafted together. The adults got into the outside catboat and watched as the kids and John followed. How Kara was going to descend the rickety ramp down fifteen feet to the dock was beyond me. But it was not beyond John. He and Tom got Kara on John's back, piggyback style and John backed down the ramp with Tom going down first spotting him just in case John slipped. Once on the dock Kara maneuvered herself into the boat and looked right at home sitting by the rail as Margie and her sister Sarah, Emily and Julia with Julia's boyfriend Sam in tow, settled in around her. John took the tiller and joined us out on the river.

We had a good steady wind and sailed in tandem, occasionally crossing tacks through the afternoon. Joanna was in charge of the adults' boat being as experienced as John at handling the catboat's huge sail and knowing the local waters. The majority of the time Maryann was at the tiller. The joke was the more Maryann talked, the worse she sailed and our sail luffed more than once while she had the helm. The storytelling and laughing was almost constant.

A definite luff, nearly into irons, occurred when Maryann was relating her story about going to see Joel Cutler for her own cardiac evaluation. With Kara out of the hospital and doing well at home for a month it had seemed appropriate for Maryann to get her cardiac status checked. She was saying that she felt a little trepidation about this visit worrying it might mean she needed a cardiac catheterization or something worse when Tom interrupted with, "So she went out and brought a new bra for the occasion." "Tom!" Maryann exclaimed. "With underwires," Tom continued, and the catboat went up into the wind. Maryann quickly recovered herself but not our course, to say, "And then I didn't even have to undress for his examination!" Our boat was almost dead in the water by this time but no one seemed to care for all the laughing. This is how it went for most of the afternoon. The kids were having just as much fun in the other boat with John's storytelling. His dog Jib jumped overboard in the middle of a tack twice. Then, when pulled back on board, he shook himself in the middle of the cockpit, soaking John and the kids.

Once, when I was leaning on the lee rail not really listening to what was going on in our boat, we crossed tacks with the kids' boat. As I caught Kara's eye, I waved and she waved back in the only way she was capable—a stiff, disjointed and mildly dystonic movement. It struck me she was slightly cut off from the kids and the rest of us by her movements and speech despite being in the midst of all our hilarity on this one in a million Maine day on the New Meadows River.

This juxtaposition put me in mind of my son Ken's senior honors paper in college. It was about a series of paintings from the seventeenth and eighteenth centuries that had been reinterpreted by a contemporary artist. Ken is interested in modern art because often it is as much about philosophy as it is about painting or sculpture. The original paintings depicted a pastoral scene from literature in which a pair of shepherds wandering in the beautiful landscape of Arcadia come on a sarcophagus with a human skull sitting on it. The words "Et in Arcadia Ego" were prominently displayed under the oversized skull and there was a look of shock on the shepherd's faces. The intent of the painting was clearly to translate the ancient Latin as if Death is speaking directly to the shepherds and to the viewer saying, "I am also in Arcadia."

This proved too direct for other artists and over time renditions of this painting softened the message by removing the skull. This allowed the shepherds and the viewer to see the scene and translate the words on the sarcophagus as if they were coming from someone who had preceded them in Arcadia and was saying, "I, once, was also in Arcadia," suggesting that whoever this person was had also enjoyed the beauty and peace of Arcadia. This allowed the viewers to reflect on this person in a happier time and skip the message about our mortality.

The point of Ken's paper was to describe Ian Hamilton Finlay's interpretation of this painting, which in an entirely different medium attempted to put back the shock of the shepherds coming on the skull. Finlay, a Scottish artist, had produced an elaborate garden around his home. In the midst of a pond with lush floral borders sat a stone model of an aircraft carrier. Around a corner in the garden path the muzzle of a German Panzer tank jutted out. Numerous other examples of modern weapons and pastoral setting existed in his garden. Ken summed up the point of what Finlay had done by writing it was the artist's intent that we should see the truth of our mortality and find ways of living with it. The message, according to Ken's paper, was to not pretend this most important fact about our lives did not exist. Since a lot of what I do is to remind people of this hard-to-face fact, I was impressed that my son had gotten this idea down by his senior year of college.

As we sailed that afternoon and Kara waved, I saw the solution to the painful truth of "Et in Arcadia Ego" emphatically symbolized by our little group in two small boats. We need each other to buffer ourselves against the terrible biologic fact of our lives. I knew Maryann and Tom knew this truth, and I felt Kara had the idea as well.

A week before this sail at the Van Ordens I had apologized to the Anglims for acting like their doctor again by asking them to get their blood drawn, so we could send it to Dr. Keating's genetics lab to be tested for the Long QT syndrome genes. We all had been enjoying Kara's being out of the hospital, and I had brought this up after a meeting where plans were being made to get her back to school. Everyone was trying to move on. I felt sad bringing them back to thoughts of Kara's Long QT syndrome and their own risk since it is a dominant trait. Maryann said I should not worry because as she said, "It is who we are now," and smiled. I never really had any doubts about this wonderful family as they went through Kara's crisis but that sentence told me why. And so on that beautiful afternoon on the New Meadows River, Maryann and Tom in our boat and Kara in the kids' boat, sailed on.

CHAPTER 25

Letters to Colleges

தை தை தை

An event is described as bittersweet when it is both happy and sad, when it is both pleasant and painful, when both good results and hard to handle results occur simultaneously. Two high school seniors who have cared for Kara since she got sick were so much changed by this experience that they used her story for their college essays. It was a bittersweet way for them to explain their feelings. Margie sent this essay to Dartmouth. She wished to write about how someone copes with a tragedy and she used me as her example.

WHEN HAIR RIBBONS MATCHED SOCKS

Maryann was standing at the end of the hallway, her face becoming clearer as I walked closer to her. I thought she would be crying, or pacing, or at least distracted. Maryann was none of these things. "Hi, Margie," she said, "How are you?" I gave her a weak smile. She seemed slightly shaken, but smiled nonetheless. Maryann is tall with short, dark hair and a round, friendly face, even when a disaster has struck. "Now I want you to know," she warned in her usual kind voice, "you can't cry in front of Kara, so get your crying out now."

This was the first of many occasions on which I realized just what kind of a person Maryann is. Her fourteen-year-old daughter, Kara, had been at track practice when Maryann was called at home and told that Kara had collapsed while she was running. Kara had been taken to Maine Medical Center and several painful hours passed before Tom and Maryann were assured that Kara would live and had some chance of recovering from brain damage. From that day forward Maryann has been patient, encouraging, determined, strong-minded and proud of Kara. Again and again Maryann has taken care of millions of problems, making millions of decisions. She has not only been a problem solver, but she has also understood something about Kara that goes beyond medical terms and everyday needs.

Surrounding the daily caloric intake chart and the physical therapy time schedule were the photos from last summer, cards, flowers and balloons. In the midst of all of these Maryann sat on the edge of the crib-like bed, softly patting Kara's leg as she explained to us that the doctors suspected that Kara had Long QT syndrome which caused her heart to go into ventricular fibrillation. Meanwhile Kara's leg kept stretching out and jerking back. Her head fell repeatedly to the left and Maryann helped her lift it back up so Kara's dazed blue eyes could see us again. For weeks Maryann massaged the spastic muscles of Kara's crumpled legs and arms and wiped the drool off her cheek. She was charmed by Kara's learning to cross her legs and excited by Kara's mumbling "Hi," her first word. "Kara, show them how you can touch your tongue to your nose," Maryann said and watched with as much pride as if Kara had just won the 100-yard backstroke as she had done a month ago.

As children my sister and I used to go to Kara's house every morning before school to wait for the bus. Once again I am going to Kara's house to help her walk into school. Instead of worrying about whether Kara's hair ribbons matched her socks, Maryann worries about whether Kara has eaten enough calories for breakfast, if Kara has had all her pills, and if Tom has brushed her teeth yet or should she. Maryann has changed from letting Kara go places alone with friends to taking her to the bathroom again, from being proud of her eighth grade report card to being excited when Kara moved up to a third grade level of reading, and from watching her daughter laugh and dance and sing to watching her struggle for minutes to get one bite of food into her mouth on her own. We're all proud of the progress Kara has made because we can see it clearly; it's harder to see how wonderful Maryann has been.

I have known Maryann for a long time, but it wasn't

125

until this unfortunate accident happened that I realized what an unusual person she is. Maryann is courageous, cheerful, clear-headed and hopeful. As I spend afternoons and lunch classes with Kara, I often ask myself if I would be able to keep smiling the way Maryann does. I'd like to think that I would.

What is interesting is I don't see myself as anything special. I see myself as doing what any parent would do in a similar situation. What I know about Margie is that she does have the strength to keep smiling through adversity. When her cardiac problem began to manifest itself and Margie was pulled from both the track team and the swim team, two of her favorite activities, she never became despondent. She trusted her doctors, trusted their treatment and now is back on the track and in the pool. And she never did stop smiling.

Sarah, Margie's sister, chose to write about the Bath community and its response to our needs in her college essays for the University of Vermont. Everything that she says in her essay is true and it shows that our family didn't make it through this experience all on our own. It was hard to feel so "needy" and to allow others to give so generously to us, knowing that we could never pay back what had been given to us. But as one friend told me, "It helps us as much as it helps you," so with that thought I was better able to accept all the gracious kindnesses shown to our family.

THROUGH AND THROUGH

On April 7, 1995, Kara Anglim went to junior high track practice as any young, dedicated runner would. She and a friend started a mile warmup, Kara chattering the whole way as usual. About halfway through the second lap, Kara stopped talking and running for a moment; a terrified look crossed her face as her lips mouthed the word, "Oh, no!" Seconds later she collapsed onto the ground, unconscious, not breathing. Seven minutes later an ambulance roared through the dirt parking lot, unsettling the dirt track as its wheels spun, digging and screaming in agony as each second threatened to take Kara's life. EMTs applied CPR and voltage to her heart and still Kara took only one breath on her own as she was quickly loaded into the ambulance. That night at the hospital, doctors told Kara's family that she had experienced Sudden Death. Her heart had gone into ventricular fibrillation. Any medical book will tell you that there is about a one percent survival rate when this happens to the heart. Kara was more than lucky—she was a miracle. The days immediately following Kara's accident were shaky. She remained in a stuporous state for two weeks. Her parents stayed by her side throughout the months she remained in the hospital, putting their own lives aside. Everyday her condition improved. First she moved her legs and then one day she smiled. These small signs of life brought hope not only to family and friends, but also to the community.

Realizing what a traumatic experience this was for Kara's family, the community of Bath, Maine took action. The first thing people did was to organize a food web so that everyday of the week all the Anglim meals were made by someone from the community. Kara's mom did not have to cook for four months. For those months, food was stacked on counters, squeezed into the refrigerator and cupboards overflowed with community support.

Days went by. The grass grew and the sheriff dropped by with his lawn mower to cut it while his son pulled weeds out of the garden. Juice and butter supplies ran low, so strangers took trips to the grocery store, then put the food in the Anglim refrigerator. Every so often Kara's family would come home from a long day at the hospital to find a friendly note carefully placed on the kitchen table. The person responsible for cleaning the house would explain they "had some extra time, and oh, by the way, I have the dog at my house, she's fine. Holler when you need her."

Walking into Kara's hospital room, just days after her accident, the walls and bulletin boards were blazing with get well cards. Over the months pictures of friends and family began to creep onto the walls and filled the spaces of the cream-colored hospital walls. Many of Kara's cards were from friends and relatives, but more than half of them were from concerned community members. On the windowsill

127

Kara's favorite type of flower, sunflowers, stood proudly; orange and yellow petals soaked the sun's rays into their thick brilliant bodies.

From the very first day of her hospitalization when rumors flew around the city about what actually had happened, Kara Anglim had and still has a support system of not only family and friends, but community. Support from the community was there through the Fourth of July when friends gathered around Kara to watch the parade, through the first night spent in her own bed at home in four months, through the first day of her high school career which began a month after all her friends had started, through trick-or-treating or taking her first step all over again. This community realized that small chores, such as taking out the garbage, or washing the dishes, were completely insignificant compared to what Kara is tackling, and so, as a community the people of Bath, Maine braided their hearts together and helped to build the bridge the Anglims had yet to cross.

A community requires involvement by all, whether that community is as small as a group of friends or a sports team, or as immense as New York City. Some communities require more time and effort from the people living within it, naturally, but if heart, generosity and kindness are opened up to others in order to make a better place, then the community and the individual will improve slowly but surely. Kara is still improving and is feeling encouragement and hope from the whole community as she trudges her way through the road to a full recovery. Realizing that a family within their community was distressed, the people of Bath are involved and helping the Anglims push onward through the deepest of trenches as Kara's recovery inches forward every day.

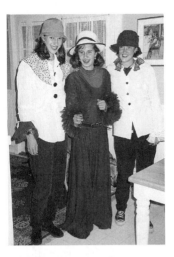

Margie and Sarah dress Kara up for a 1995 Halloween party.

CHAPTER 26

Changes

by Walter Allan, M.D.

❦ ❦ ❦

There have been changes for Tom, Maryann and Guerin just as there have been changes for Kara. What the lack of oxygen and blood flow to Kara's brain did to her can readily be seen by anyone. What it did to each of her family members is much harder to see. How Kara will look, act and talk a year and more from now is not possible to know. So it is impossible to write the final chapter of Kara's story. But certain things are true about Kara now and will be true about her a year from now. That is, she is still the same wonderful, determined, funny person she was before her cardiac arrest. We see evidence of that daily in the things she says and the way she works at her rehabilitation. And her family remains the same wonderful, determined, funny group they were before this happened. This book is ample evidence of that.

As for changes in each of the Anglims, there are the obvious and the not so obvious. Their schedule revolves around Kara and her needs. All family activities have to take into account what Kara can and cannot do. Mostly these are minor inconveniences, but it is easy to see how their home life has dramatically changed from what it was before April 7, 1995. Then there are the personal changes I do not know but can guess at from the stories I hear.

Once in February 1996, Kara stopped in the middle of reading a story with Maryann and started to cry. She said it was because she knew she used to be able to do things like reading so much more easily. It was one of the few times Kara cried since she left the hospital. After Maryann told me that story, I asked Kara during a private moment together if she felt sad at times. She said "Yes." I asked what she thought about when she was sad, thinking I could reassure her about her continuing recovery. But her answer surprised me. Instead of thoughts about her own recovery she said that her sadness usually involved thoughts about Jesse. He was the boy in the next room at Maine Medical Center. He was a patient of mine with torsion dystonia who became Kara's friend in the hospital. I am sure Kara recognized his suffering and his kindness and, perhaps, she saw similarities in their neurologic predicaments.

Maryann's stories have to do with the trouble she has going out in public because of the people she is likely to run into and the painful questions she will have to answer. But in her typical fashion, she sees humor in this situation. She says it affects what her family eats. Recently, on a trip to the grocery store she was planning a stew but there were too many people she knew shopping in the vegetable section, so the family got chili since the canned kidney bean aisle was clear.

Tom meets the public daily in his practice as a dentist and does not have the luxury of darting down the kidney bean aisle. Tom's stories are about how he has learned to deflect questions concerning Kara with minimal replies and a new joke. I have heard lots of jokes from Tom and all of them are funnier than the "termite" joke.

I know least about how these changes affected Guerin. She has been away at college and struggling through the usual first year adjustments. Maryann tells me Guerin talks to Kara on the phone from school when she is at school and takes her shopping when she is home on vacation. These times with Guerin, Maryann says, are Kara's biggest thrill. But since Guerin is away from the family much of the time she has had less time to talk all of this through. However, I suspect Guerin, like the rest of her family, realizes she has the inner strength to meet life's crises head-on and endure the changes they bring.

I would never have predicted the changes I have seen in myself over the months since Kara was admitted to Maine Medical Center. What I did as a doctor for the Anglims, I intend to do for all my patients and their families. It just does not happen that often that I can play such a personal role. Partly this is because of who I am and partly it is because of who they are. But it does happen from time to time that a family will let you answer all their questions and listen at the same time. If you all have similar philosophies of life and the patient's problems are serious enough, you get to be an important part of their lives. I can count on my fingers how many times this has happened to me in eighteen years in practice in Maine. What has never happened before is a friendship such as I have developed with the Anglims. It came about partly because I was on sabbatical.

I had arranged a six-month sabbatical at a local research lab. I told Maryann about it when I saw Kara for the last time in my office a month before her cardiac arrest. Maryann, jokingly, asked me to promise to take care of Kara while I was on sabbatical and I, jokingly, said I would. She reminded me of this promise about a month after Kara was hospitalized. I decided not to go back on that promise and it ended up doing more for me than it did for Kara.

The reason for my sabbatical was partly to see if I could do things I had done decades before as a biochemistry graduate student and partly to escape medicine. There is too much whining in the daily practice of medicine, at least the outpatient medicine I was doing. At first, I thought the whining was coming from my fellow doctors and from disgruntled patients, but since I am back doing the same job in the same office and do not notice it as much, I wonder if the whining might not actually have come from me. I remember I began to notice less of it back before I actually left for my sabbatical. This coincided with my twice daily visits to see Kara. I got involved with the Anglims and making sure things worked as well as possible while Kara healed. In the hospital they needed me to do this, but they also wanted me to do this, and finally, they let me do it.

While on sabbatical, I had more time for things they no longer needed me to do, but some they let me do anyway. Early in the fall, after Kara left the hospital, I arranged to take her home each Monday after her rehabilitation appointment in Portland. I would pick Kara up and drive the forty-five minutes to Bath so neither Tom nor Maryann had to make that trip twice in one day. My wife saw how important this was to me and joined Kara, Maryann, Tom and me for dinners filled with fast-paced conversation and high hilarity on those nights. This helped seal the friendship between our two families.

The end result of this experience for me is a reaffirmation of my idea of what it is to be a doctor. Although I never expect to form such a friendship with a family again, I learned through my experience with Kara the value of the important little things I do as a doctor—to listen patiently and to allow the families realistic hope whenever possible. I set out on my sabbatical to see if I could change who I am and ended up the same old guy but, importantly, without the whining. I did change who I am to a certain extent. I think of myself now as an uncle. I have taken to calling myself Uncle Walter with Kara as Ann and I have grown closer to the Anglims. I figure it is probably good to have at least one crazy uncle per family and I am trying hard to fill that role. I wonder if this might be more difficult than just being her doctor.

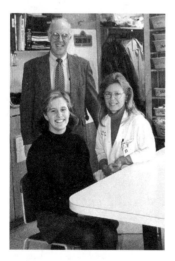

Kara, Dr. Bagwell and Dr. Allan, Christmas 1996
(Uncle Walter never wears a suit).

CHAPTER 27

A Thousand Cranes

৬ঌ৬ঌ৬ঌ

Right before Kara collapsed in April 1995, we had a Japanese exchange student stay with us for a short visit. Her name was Ayako and she was Kara's age. She had come to Maine with a group of her classmates and they were attending school with their host brothers and sisters and experiencing American food and culture. Mostly, they were having a lot of fun despite the obvious language difference. In February 1996 a package arrived in the mail from Ayako. We opened it to find a beautiful and colorful origami mobile consisting of a thousand cranes. The note to Kara said:

Dear Kara,
Hello, I am Ayako. Do you remember me? I was surprised to learn that you were in the hospital. But you are in the house, aren't you? I am very much concerned about your health. I hope you will get well soon. This is thousand cranes. We call them "senbazuru." Japanese people make a thousand cranes when someone becomes sick. Why we make a thousand cranes? Because, to wish for them recovery. This was made by my family, my friends and me. Smile.
Ayako

I knew the story of *Sadako and the Thousand Paper Cranes* by Eleanor Coerr. It is a book about a Japanese girl, a runner, who dies of leukemia. There was a mobile of a thousand cranes in the playroom of the Pediatric Unit at the Maine Medical Center. I had studied it often as I tried to imagine for whom it had been made. And now Kara had her own one thousand cranes, made with love and sent many miles across many cultures with the messages of health and recovery.

Maybe it was the thousand cranes which helped Kara in her earliest days of speech therapy when she was still safety-strapped into her wheelchair and she struggled to recall the words to identify the simplest objects such as a ball or a brush. Despite her language impairment and dystonia, she still kept her sense of humor. When Susan, the speech therapist, taped Kara using a video camera and microphone, Kara would eye the camera, grab the microphone and sing different tones. As soon as Susan turned her back, Kara would bend down to the microphone, look up at the camera and say "Hi, Mom." Susan once asked Kara to identify five different fruits, and Kara tried to get away with saying: "Apple, banana, banana, banana, banana." Of course, Susan wouldn't let her off that easily and when she gave her appropriate hints, Kara did produce the words for five different fruits. One was blueberries, and when Susan asked Kara if she liked blueberries, she said, "Yuk, hate them." Her teenage likes and dislikes were definitely present. Now her speech is still slightly slow and thick, but she can easily communicate every need. When we have a hard time understanding a particular word or phrase, Kara patiently spells it for us.

Maybe it was the thousand cranes which helped Kara through her feeding difficulties. Kara had always been a picky eater and now she was worse. Feeding Kara orally was a time-consuming frustrating chore. She would store the food in her mouth for many minutes only to spit it out when we realized that she hadn't talked for a while. Once on the Pediatric Unit I thought I had done a good job of feeding Kara and left her room for a few minutes to visit the mother of Kara's next door neighbor. When I came back in the room, there was Dr. Allan holding a styrofoam cup full of Kara's half-digested food. "Oops", I said, "I guess that I forgot something." It is good practice for neurologists to have to deal with this sort of thing. Now her eating is so much better. She even eats broccoli and spinach and seems to have weaned herself from Skittles, her usual food of choice.

Maybe it was the thousand cranes which helped Kara through her severe dystonia. There were days that Tom didn't come home until one or two o'clock in the morning as he tried to soothe Kara through her sleepless dystonic episodes. He would walk her around the hospital halls all evening trying to tire her out. He would sing to her and rub her back as he tried to get her to settle down for a night of slumber. He would come home distraught from watching our daughter pass through this restless and seemingly physically painful period. He felt helpless. But now she falls off to sleep easily each night, all snug and comfy in a bed listening to her favorite tapes. When Guerin first took Kara swimming for her recreational therapy, it would take forever for her to wiggle Kara into her bathing suit as she pried her arms and legs into the appropriate openings. Now Kara is progressing towards dressing herself.

Maybe it was the thousand cranes which helped Kara make the adjustment to school. She started school in October but her endurance was so low that she could barely make it through the day. Her attention span was short and ability to focus on tasks limited. But slowly she got better. Now at the end of a school day she still had the energy to climb the last flight of stairs up to the art room or to go to the YMCA for a swim therapy session. She took speech and chorus with her classmates. She went into regular classes when they had projects that she was capable of doing. I help her with special projects—I now know as much as most astronomers about the winter sky. Her math is at a sixth-grade level and some of her verbal skills are already beyond her age level. People are starting to see not a child to be pitied but a child to be honored for her courage and commitment to recovery.

Maybe it was the thousand cranes which sent Margie and Sarah, Emily and Julia to Kara. Kara is extremely sociable and loves people. Margie and Sarah are the two wonderful people who make sure that Kara's social needs are met. They take her to basketball games, shopping and out for ice cream. If they are with her for meals, they patiently encourage her eating and even feed her. They were her dates to the high school's winter dance and told her how beautiful she looked in her short, little black dress with her black tights and her Doc Marten shoes. They made sure that she never had one lonely moment that night. I don't think that they have any idea what a huge part of Kara's recovery they are. I try to spoil them every chance that I get, but I don't think that I will ever be able to repay all that they have done for our family. Emily and Julia are identical blond blue-eyed twins. They watch over Kara's academic career. It is Emily who is reading Roald Dahl's *Matilda* with Kara and it was Julia's suggestion to the teacher that placed Kara in a regular speech class. One day Emily asked Kara, "Is speech your favorite class?" Kara answered back to her friend, "Emily, it is my only class!" There is nothing wrong with Kara's sense of humor.

Maybe it was the thousand cranes which have made our home life a little easier with each passing day. Having Kara with us at home is a privilege but there is no doubt that our lives have changed dramatically. We still cannot leave Kara home alone because if there were a fire or if someone came to the door, she couldn't reliably handle the situation. We still have to bathe her, help dress her, help her feed herself and entertain her. But it is easier to do all of these chores than when she first came home in July 1995, and she contributes more to her own care each day.

Everything we do with her we approach as a rehab opportunity because we want to utilize every moment to aid her healing. We read to her and with her, do crossword puzzles together, help create bold Matisse-like paintings, practice using the computer and play games with her. We try to plan family outings that will be both fun and therapeutic for her. All of this takes energy and time and what suffers are those moments every adult so enjoys, the time to read as you listen to music, the time to build our kayak, and the time for Tom and me to rent a movie and enjoy it together. Now by the time nine o'clock rolls around every night, Tom and I are barely able to keep our eyes open. But every day there is a reward, either in what Kara says or what she does. That is what keeps us motivated and lets us know that a day will come when we will smile at each other and know that we did our best for our daughter.

So those thousand cranes are doing their job. Those prayers that you pray for Kara in your Buddhist temples are a testament to the commonality of our human spirits and we are humbly grateful. Thank you, Ayako, Shuji, Asuka, Katsuya, Mizuki, Hirokazu, Hidetoki, Futoshi, Koji, Daiki, Shoichi, Sayaka, Erika K., Reina, Jurika, Yuka, Mayu, Sayuri, Mikako, Asuka, Chinatsu, Yuki, Yuka, Rika, Erika N. and Kazuko.

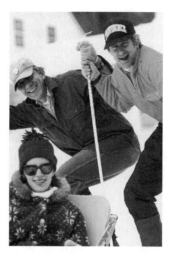

John Van Orden and Tom take Kara for a sled ride in December 1995.

CHAPTER 28

Getting Dizzy

❧ ❧ ❧

Part I

I grew up in a neighborhood full of children in a suburb of Chicago. When I was a little girl, my friends and I had many summer days filled with nothing but games. Our favorite was getting dizzy. We would spin ourselves around and around on someone's lawn until we were so dizzy that we would fall over, and then we would open our eyes and watch the world spin around us. The game was even better if we had dresses on because then we fancied ourselves resembling big spinning flowers. Probably all the boys in the neighborhood were there looking at our underwear, but we were too naive to notice. As we grew older, we were allowed to walk to the park where we would twist the chains on the swings around as tightly as they would go, sit down on the swing's seat and then spin out of control as simultaneously we swung as high and fast as we could possibly go. When the spin was over, we would catapult ourselves from the swing and fly into the air out as far as gravity would allow us. Getting dizzy was a lot of fun.

But for Kara getting dizzy is not fun. Getting dizzy scares her incredibly because to her it means that she is going to pass out. Feeling dizzy was the final sensation she had before her cardiac arrest. The last time that Kara felt dizzy since then was February 10, 1996. She was at the YMCA with her friends, excited to be part of the swim team picture which was being taken. As Margie, Sarah and Julia walked her over to the bleachers, they felt her stumble. Margie turned to help Kara correct her balance when Kara said, "I feel dizzy." Margie real-

139

ized that something was wrong and helped Kara lie down on the floor as Julia went to get her mother and Sarah went to call 911. Kara's eyes were closed, she was shivering and shaking and suddenly her shoulder jerked. This all happened within the span of a few seconds. By the time that Julia's mother, my friend Linda, and my friend John Van Orden knelt beside Kara, she was awake and oriented although her color was pale but dusky around her lips. "Did I pee myself?" she whispered to Linda, because that had happened once before when she had passed out. "No," Linda said, "but I almost did."

Kara was crying and scared. Then she overheard that the ambulance was coming to take her to the emergency room in Bath. The tears started in earnest until the EMT walked in and she saw it was Alan Douglass, the same person who had resuscitated her with David Hudson at the track. She said, "I'm not scared anymore." Magically, the tears stopped. It probably helped that Alan is a tall, cute, red-headed guy.

Linda rode with Kara in the ambulance to the hospital and John called me at home from the YMCA to tell me in his calm and reassuring "doctor voice" what had happened. "She is fine now," he assured me, "so don't worry." But, of course, I had to worry a little. By the time I got to the emergency room, Sarah and Margie, John and Linda were all gathered around Kara as she ate a sprinkled cupcake while lying on the emergency room stretcher hooked up to the ECG monitor. My family is used to having me make a joke about most everything. John and Linda have the same sense of humor so I'm sure that Kara thought she was a part of a stand-up comedy routine as we cracked jokes while simultaneously assessing the monitor, her color, her ability to cerebrate, her oxygen saturation and her blood pressure.

John called Dr. Cutler's office, explained the situation to him and asked if we could fax Kara's ECG down to him in Portland. "We are not leaving this emergency room until we fax Kara's ECG down to Joel Cutler and have him assess it," said John, now in his take-charge-doctor-mode. "This is the '90s and we are going to use the technology." I might have eventually arrived at this decision myself, but John saw it more quickly. Soon Joel was on the telephone with me, assuring me that Kara was now fine, that she could be discharged from the emergency room, that her ECG looked normal for her with all of her paced ventricular beats, and that if I needed him, all I had to do was beep him.

Every three months, Kara goes for a routine visit to Joel's office and he evaluates the function of her defibrillator/pacemaker as he places a "wand" over the device. Does that sound magical? It should, because it is. Not only does the monitor display her current ECG, it also tells how many times the device has paced and defibrillated over the past three months and the current energy status of the battery. Kara's device has defibrillated her twice, once in October 1995 and once on February 10, 1996. During her November visit, Joel told me that Kara had gone into ventricular fibrillation and the device had delivered a shock that had returned her heart to a normal rhythm on a Wednesday evening in October at 7:15 p.m. I was totally surprised because Kara had neither reported a peculiar feeling to me nor had I noticed anything unusual. At that point in her recuperative phase, she would often go to bed at 7:00 p.m, so I think I wasn't with her when it happened.

It was hard for me to hear that Kara had experienced another "event" as the doctors tend to call these episodes. It was a reminder that she did, indeed, have a serious and life-threatening heart syndrome. It shook my stability. But Joel must have known that because he was so positive. "This is great," he said, "because now we have a definite diagnosis. We know we did the right thing. We know the defibrillator works the way we had hoped." He was actually happy. He gave me a hug and said, "Everything is fine." That made me smile in a resigned sort of way. I knew that once again, I would readjust my paradigms, and adopt his attitude as my attitude. After this first defibrillation, he put her on 50 milligrams of a beta-blocking medication called atenolol and after the second defibrillation, he upped the dosage to 100 milligrams. Since then, she has had no further incidents of ventricular fibrillation.

This is Tom's and my reality, and this is what we live with every day. How do we do it? I'll give you the simple key which is in a verse that someone quoted to me:

A BAG OF TOOLS
By R.L. Sharpe

Isn't it strange
That princes and kings,
And clowns that caper
In sawdust rings,
And common people
Like you and me
Are builders for eternity?

Each is given a bag of tools,
A shapeless mass,
A set of rules;
And each must make-
Ere life is flown-
A stumbling block
Or a steppingstone.

I guess that it is obvious that Tom, Guerin, Kara and I fashioned a steppingstone.

Getting Dizzy

৩ ৩ ৩

Part II
by Walter Allan, M.D.

When Maryann and Kara visited Joel Cutler's office in March, the stored event retrieved from Kara's ICD showed the dizzy spell in February had been another episode of ventricular fibrillation. This is a copy of that episode:

The strip should be read from left to right. At the bot-

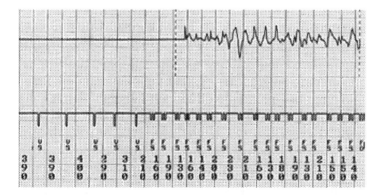

tom of the strip you see numbers printed vertically. These are beat-to-beat intervals in milliseconds. That is, the time between each successive heartbeat is measured in thousands of a second and stored by the ICD. An interval of 390 milliseconds converts to a heart rate of 154. Thus, at the beginning of this strip Kara's heart had sped up considerably. When the beat-to-beat interval reached 140 to 200 milliseconds, or more than 300 beats per minute, the ICD stored the actual ECG as shown above the numbers. This tracing confirms ventricular fibrillation. Just following the trace of ECG (not shown) the ICD delivered a shock that converted Kara's heartbeat back to normal.

How and why Kara's heartbeat went from its usual regular pace to this pattern is not known. The theory is that somehow the next heartbeat comes too soon for the heart muscle to conduct normally. Maybe this happened in February because of all the excitement Kara experienced being with her swim team for the first time since her cardiac arrest. In any event, it is felt that this early beat arrives in a portion of the heart muscle that is still in what is called the "vulnerable period." This is the period of time when the muscle cells are becoming repolarized. The cells are recharging their membranes in order to generate another regular contraction. This is the portion of a heartbeat that represents most of the time measured by the QT interval. Even though Kara does not consistently have a measurably prolonged QT interval, she has shown repeatedly that she must have an increased vulnerable period allowing an early beat to produce the disastrous change in heart rhythm that is ventricular fibrillation. Without her implantable cardiac defibrillator, Kara would not be with us. It is as simple as that.

The event in February was witnessed and, perhaps, Alan Douglass could have gotten there in time once again. But the event in October occurred while Kara was alone in her room, without warning or observers, and would have killed her without the ICD's countershock. Joel Cutler has told me that some of his patients have a lot of trouble living with that idea. They have a horrible dread of the dizziness that portends their events and the feel of the countershock. Some of his patients live minute-to-minute with this dread and sense of foreboding. Kara and her family have accepted this possibility with the same courage, trust and hope that has characterized their approach to the rest of Kara's story.

CHAPTER 29

What Does It Mean to have a Gene?
by Walter Allan, M.D.

੭ ੭ ੭

More than a year after we had sent the blood samples on Kara, Guerin, Tom and Maryann to Dr. Mark Keating's lab in Salt Lake City we still did not have the results. This is not a problem with Dr. Keating's lab, but rather is a problem with DNA testing in general. Because the Keating lab is in the process of discovering the mutations associated with Long QT syndrome and working out how these mutations produce their effects, they can only test the most informative samples. In order to identify the DNA link with a disease the blood samples of at least eight affected and eight unaffected family members are needed. Thus, larger family groups than the Anglims would be screened first.

This problem is not unique to Long QT syndrome. Although new gene mutations that are responsible for inherited diseases are being discovered at a tremendous rate, tests for these mutations do not easily become available in the day-to-day practice of medicine. Partly this is because these tests are still in the research phase when they are announced and the full ramifications of having a specific mutation have not been worked out. And partly it is in the nature of genetic tests in general. This brings up the question of how could knowing the results of DNA tests be of help to the Anglims?

Our hypothesis was that Kara and Maryann had one of the previously discovered mutations (or perhaps, a unique mutation) in one of the ion channel genes. Testing could have confirmed that. Testing could also have excluded Tom as the

145

originator of the gene in Kara. And, finally, it would have been good news for the Anglims if the testing had shown that Guerin did not have the gene. Until Dr. Keating's lab found a mutation accounting for Kara's Long QT syndrome which could be excluded in Guerin, Guerin would have to be considered at risk for sudden death. This was true even though Guerin had a normal QT interval on her ECG because a small percentage of people with a Long QT syndrome gene will have a normal QT interval. Guerin is on a swimming scholarship at Providence College and since the provocative event that produces ventricular fibrillation in individuals with Long QT Syndrome is often high-level exercise, Maryann and Tom could not help but worry about her fifty percent risk of having the gene. As with other autosomal dominant conditions, we think we know what it means to NOT have the gene. The person is NOT at increased risk of the family's inherited condition. But what if Guerin had the gene? And what does it mean that Maryann has the gene?

A germ line (or inherited) mutation in a cardiac ion channel gene alters cells in every person who has that mutation. However, not every person with this alteration suffers the consequences of having abnormal cardiac repolarization to the degree that Kara did. Maryann, for instance, has had only a single fainting episode that she can recall, but that occurred under emotional circumstances. Since a single fainting episode is quite frequent in people in general and has many benign causes, that single episode for Maryann may not have been a result of the characteristic ventricular tachycardia that occurs in Long QT syndrome. However, knowing with the certainty of DNA testing that Maryann has the gene and that this gene had the terrible consequences that it did for Kara, it makes sense to protect Maryann. A daily dose of a beta-blocker—a drug that prevents a rapid heartbeat by blocking the sympathetic nervous system input to the heart—is very effective protection. Mike Vincent told me he has never had a patient die who was adequately beta-blocked. Maryann decided to go on a beta-blocker when we recognized she had a prolonged QT interval, so the gene test would not have altered what we did for

Maryann. If Guerin had the gene, I would have advocated she also take a beta-blocker. But since she had never had an episode, Guerin may have objected to the treatment. What then? What risk would Guerin be facing?

This is where our scientific knowledge begins to show its weakness, the same weakness we hoped would be remedied by finding the genetic basis of Long QT syndrome. Having the gene does not mean the affected person will suffer a cardiac arrest or even faint. This is called variability of expression and is common in autosomal dominant disorders. Why that is, is not known. It may be because other altered genes are needed for the problem to be as serious as it was in Kara. Or it may have to do with something else about the person or their environment. For instance, the serum potassium can drop from a variety of causes and make the person with Long QT syndrome more susceptible to problems with cardiac ion channels. We had such a case this past summer. A child presented to our emergency room because of a faint or seizure. He was visiting Maine from Utah and had become dehydrated on a hot summer day. The serum potassium was low and the ECG showed a prolonged QT interval. Dick McFaul, the pediatric cardiologist who first evaluated Kara, saw the child and recognized this association since he had just read a paper about Long QT syndrome and low potassium. He wrote a letter to the child's physician in Utah and mentioned Dr. Vincent as a resource.

There could be other reasons that the gene expresses itself more dramatically as well. When Dick McFaul saw Kara at age eight, he pointed out that Kara had a will that exceeded her endurance when she did her treadmill test. Could that have had something to do with Kara's multiple episodes of what we thought were seizures? There has always been a theory that the nervous system plays a role in the events associated with the gene for Long QT syndrome. Why else would exercise or being startled by an alarm clock be associated with attacks? Could it be that if Kara had a different personality, she would not have had a cardiac arrest? This same drive is what we love about her and is what is carrying her through and getting her better despite her cardiac arrest. Should we wish (for wishing is all we can do about it) that Kara had a different personality? It reminds me of the comment Maryann made to me when I worried that I was reminding them of Kara's problem as we left the first pupil evaluation team meeting in fall 1995. "It is who we are," was what she said, and I think she would say the same thing if I asked her that question about Kara's personality.

Convincing people that Long QT syndrome is a real threat can be difficult. It goes against our common sense notion of our own health. People with Long QT syndrome feel fine. It is not until someone in their family suffers a cardiac arrest that the terrible nature of this condition becomes evident. Some families with Long QT syndrome will have a low mortality rate per affected person per year and other families will have a high rate. But even a high risk of sudden death is on the order of one percent per year. That sort of information was not known by the Anglims since they have just discovered this gene in their family and as far as they can trace the family tree, no one else has had sudden death. It may turn out that the different mutations in the more than four different genes for Long QT syndrome are associated with different risks of sudden death. That is information that we do not have at present but information that could be used to convince individuals of the gravity of the problem.

Because the diagnosis is still relatively unknown and difficult to make, it can be missed even when a sudden death occurs in successive generations. This story is all too common, and our cardiologists recently referred a patient to our genetics group at the Foundation for Blood Research where I continue to work since doing my sabbatical. This patient, Mrs. Childs, had lost her brother, her daughter and then her granddaughter before Long QT syndrome was considered. Her story is instructive since it shows how insidious this condition can be and how having a test that can establish the diagnosis with certainty could be helpful.

Mrs. Childs's Story

In the winter of 1996 (about a year after Kara's arrest) our local newspaper had a story about a twelve year-old girl who died a sudden cardiac death while playing basketball on her middle school team in South Hiram, Maine. Brandy died in front of teammates, coaches and spectators. Sudden death in a young healthy person always causes a tremendous stir in a community. The report in the papers of the funeral at the school tells that story. All this publicity, however, would eventually serve this family well.

In the weeks following Brandy's death Mrs. Childs, her grandmother, kept calling the state coroner's office to find out what had caused her granddaughter to die. She was told there was no discernible cause. Brandy was cared for by her grandmother because Brandy's mother (Mrs. Childs's daughter) had dropped dead while standing in the kitchen having a cup of coffee years before. Brandy's mother had a history of drug abuse so her death had been attributed in some way to that. Mrs. Childs had never believed this since her daughter was not using drugs at the time her death occurred. In addition, Mrs. Childs's brother had driven to work one day at age forty-four and was later found dead at the wheel of his truck. He had been in good health all his life.

A few weeks after Brandy's funeral, Mrs. Childs got a phone call from an older woman she remotely knew in a neighboring town. This woman asked Mrs. Childs if she had ever heard of Long QT syndrome and when Mrs. Childs said she had not, the woman told her the story of her family. Mrs. Childs's acquaintance had lost two sons to sudden cardiac death and only recently had doctors for her other two sons discovered that their family had Long QT syndrome. The woman advised Mrs. Childs to call Brandy's doctor and ask about it. She did and Dr. Neil Korsen (a family practitioner trained at Maine Medical Center) said he had never heard of it but would find out more for her. He called Maribeth Hourihan. She told Dr. Korsen to have Mrs. Childs and her family get ECGs and to have Brandy's siblings come see her and Mrs. Childs's children see Joel Cutler.

As our cardiologists took the family history, it turned out Mrs. Childs had eleven siblings! She had four children herself and each of Mrs. Childs's brothers and sisters had children. Maribeth found prolonged QT intervals in two of Mrs. Childs's grandchildren who were Brandy's siblings and a suspicious QT in the other sibling. Joel found suspicious QTs in Brandy's uncles and aunts. They knew they had uncovered a very large kindred of Long QT syndrome and perhaps one hundred people could be at risk.

I became involved with this large family through my new position at the Foundation for Blood Research. As we took down the pedigree, I was struck by how many young adults had died of what was said to be a seizure. Mrs. Childs had a great aunt Tora who remembered her grandfather had died as a young man in a small fishing village in Denmark before her grandmother had immigrated to this country. As Mrs. Childs was in the process of rounding up information about her family tree, a friend called to tell her the *Reader's Digest* had an article about Long QT syndrome. This article discussed Mike Vincent's work with the large family of Danish descent in Utah named Christensen. That family had come to the United States about the same time Aunt Tora mentioned Mrs. Childs's ancestors had immigrated. After reading the *Reader's Digest* article Mrs. Childs asked Aunt Tora the name of her Danish grandfather who had died in a seizure, and Tora said it was Christensen. Mrs. Childs wondered if she could be related to the Long QT syndrome family Mike Vincent has helped. Interestingly, Mike Vincent told me there was a rumor that there was another Christensen brother, so it could be that Mrs. Childs's family is part of this very large Utah pedigree. We are currently trying to gather this large family in our area to screen them for the condition and place those who are affected on beta-blockers. When genetic testing on Mrs. Childs's blood sample is completed, we will know whether or not her family is a branch of this large Danish family with Long QT syndrome.

The fact that a deadly condition like this can be in a family for generations without coming to light is what makes

Long QT syndrome such a challenge. It is likely, as in Mrs. Childs's case, that public education does a better job than physician education at finding new cases and getting the correct treatment. The reason for this is that people with Long QT syndrome are largely healthy and do not see physicians. And if they do, the story of their faints might never come up. When someone dies, more common and less complex reasons are given as the cause of death unless someone knows about Long QT syndrome. But once you know about this condition, you worry that it is everywhere. Maryann cannot read a newspaper report of the sudden death of an athlete or a young person without thinking of Long QT syndrome. And every time I see someone in my office with a faint or an unexplained seizure, I see Kara sitting on my exam table telling me about seeing that blue light in March 1995. It is true for others in our community as well. Because of Kara and her story, our pediatric and adult cardiologists and neurologists are much more aware of this condition than they had been in the past.

The diagnosis is likely to remain a challenge for the near future. Gene testing is not available as a routine laboratory test at present, and new mutations are likely to be discovered which will make testing for the condition more difficult as time passes. But, these are technical problems that will eventually be worked out. More problematic is what to do when we have a technically good test and can uncover the genetic mutations in anyone tested. Who do we test? Everyone at birth? Will the mutations that cause Long QT syndrome be screened for along with multiple other mutations as part of a routine newborn infant blood test? And what other genes will also be screened?

The mutations that cause Long QT syndrome can be thought of as "susceptibility" genes. That is, they pass on to an affected person a susceptibility for the consequences of having a problem with cardiac muscle repolarization (fainting, secondary seizures or cardiac arrest). These consequences may never occur. Of course, if they do occur, and are benign, treatment could be instituted then. However, family stories of Long QT syndrome are full of examples where the first event in an affected individual is sudden death. So maybe we should decide to treat every affected individual with beta-blockers. This is not a bad solution for Long QT syndrome, since the treatment is relatively benign, although a lifetime treatment with any medicine is a problem. But what about the other "susceptibility" genes we were also going to screen? Knowing about a gene mutation where there is no treatment or the treatment is drastic is a major problem. An example is BRCA-1, the breast cancer susceptibility gene. Women who inherit a mutation in that gene face a lifetime risk of breast cancer of 85-90%. Since, statistically, breast cancer will not occur until age 30 or more, surveillance is all that is needed until that age. But then surgery to remove both breasts and ovaries may be recommended. Is this something someone wants to anticipate from birth? Hopefully, better surveillance or treatment will become available so that this drastic preventative treatment will not be necessary. But until it is, knowing about BRCA-1 is a mixed blessing.

I have learned over the past two years since Kara's cardiac arrest that it is not easy to know what it means to have a susceptibility gene. And there is a lot to work out before we can give families information to help them decide how to face their risk when a susceptibility gene is discovered. Hopefully, in the near future we will be able to tell with certainty when Long QT syndrome is present and what degree of risk that mutation confers to an affected person. But there is still much for medical science to discover to really know what it means to have a Long QT syndrome gene.

Chapter 30

"So, *how* is Kara doing, Dr. Allan?"

by Walter Allan, M.D.

↩ ↩ ↩

As months and then a year and more passed following Kara's cardiac arrest, I would still get asked how she was doing. The pediatric and intensive care nurses, therapists and social workers would stop me as I came on the ward or got on an elevator to ask about Kara. This has happened with other patients but not to the extent it has happened with Kara. Largely this is explained by how involved they all felt in Kara's care and by the special qualities everyone recognized in Kara, Maryann and Tom. But I think it is also explained by how involved they knew I was with Kara. One way they knew about that was because of Maryann's grand rounds.

In the winter following Kara's discharge, the rehabilitation department asked Carol Zechman, our social worker, to organize a grand rounds dealing with the special issues of pediatric rehabilitation. This is a weekly conference for the rehabilitation department at Maine Medical Center which includes physicians, therapists and nurses from the rehabilitation floor. Carol asked me if I thought Maryann would come and speak at the rounds. I was sure she would and told Carol about our book, *Kara Mia*. When I asked Maryann about the idea she agreed and at first thought it might be easy as she could just read sections from the book. But she also wanted somehow to show the therapists how far Kara had come thanks to them and the therapists at BaySide. We hit on the idea of showing a videotape of Kara since Kara was in the process of making a tape at BaySide to be shown to her classmates at

Morse High School. We also remembered that Sue Rhyberg, Kara's speech therapist while she was hospitalized, had taped several speech therapy sessions with Kara.

I arranged to get the tapes from Sue and together with the audio visual technician at Maine Medical Center, Maryann and I edited them. The final copy was remarkable. We picked Kara's first taped speech session in May, one in June and then a session done on the day before discharge. These were followed by the tape Kara was making at BaySide. All of Kara's hospital speech sessions showed her in a wheelchair, whereas she was walking unaided in the BaySide tape. But beyond that, Kara's total appearance changed over the time covered by these tapes. Kara was barely audible during the first session in May. Her speech sounded strained and, because of all her associated movements, it looked as if the act of speaking required a superhuman effort. Watching her great difficulties moving and speaking during that first session brought back hard memories for Maryann and me as we first reviewed the tape. But even the June speech session showed improvement and by the time the BaySide tape was made Kara looked remarkably improved. So the overall effect was one of steady recovery. But still, the tape brought out the reality of how severely affected Kara had been and still, in many ways, is.

This reality, and the act of reading her written words aloud, was more difficult than Maryann originally thought. She dealt with this by practicing her talk at home until it was so routine she thought it had all the emotion drained out of it. However, this did not prove to be quite the case when the day arrived to speak before the staff. She carried it off laughing through some tears as she had carried off so many other moments at Maine Medical Center. Tom and Kara were there, as were the Van Ordens, to support her. Carol Zechman saw to it that the pediatric nurses knew about Maryann's rounds. She read her book and played the video to a packed house. Hearing and seeing what it had meant to the Anglims to be cared for by our team was a moving experience for everyone and it blew my cover as "just the doctor." After Maryann's grand rounds everyone knew I had a special relationship with this family.

In addition, the word got out that Maryann was writing a book about this experience and I was contributing some chapters. This kept Kara's story on the minds of all those people who had worked closely with her and the Anglims. They always had questions. Early on, just after Kara left the hospital, it was easy to talk about her progress. Going from a wheelchair to walking unaided is a landmark everyone can appreciate. But as time passed, it became harder to describe her progress, and there was always a silent question lurking behind the spoken one. That question was going to be more difficult to answer. What about the future?

So what do I say when people ask how Kara is doing? Most of the time it is sufficient to say things such as, "She's doing better and better," or, "She is back at school two days a week and goes shopping at the mall with her sister, Guerin, when she's home from college." But there are some nurses, such as Carol MacVane whom I've known so long, who do not let me get away with such pat replies. Carol is someone who will ask the question behind the question. She will cast a skeptical eye at me and ask aloud what I think the future holds for Kara. She periodically asks if I think Kara will ever be "normal." "You just never know," is my offhand way of dealing with Carol's question if I can get away with it.

But it is, of course, the question to which everyone wants to know the answer—Tom and Maryann, Guerin, their friends, my family, Kara's teachers, therapists and maybe, even most of all, Kara. Only Kara and the rest of them never ask. At least not directly. But it is part of my job to try and answer this sort of question everyday. So I cannot help but ask it of myself while at the same time knowing it is impossible to answer. One of my favorite quotes on this topic comes from the Danish physicist and humanist, Neils Bohr: "Prediction, especially of the future, is difficult." As true as that statement is, it does not stop us from asking and hoping.

This mix of hope and the need for reality often get muddled in my office as I found the other day in a conversation with the mother of a seven year old girl with a very bad

epilepsy and autism. She was asking about some minor seizures her daughter was having and was quite discouraged by
the fact that the seizures had not completely gone away. I was
trying to emphasize the fact that her major seizures had not
occurred in quite awhile and she was actually doing better.
When we got close to understanding each other I ended the
conversation by saying in my kindest way, "You know from all
you have been through, that Stephanie is not really ever going
to be much different than she is today." And then realizing
what I had just said I added, "But I don't want you to give up
hope, now."

I am much less certain of an answer in Kara's case and
there is no question of giving up hope, but what will be her
reality? After Kara's first few months out of the hospital the
big landmarks of improvement had been accomplished. She
was walking alone and looked less and less stiff in moving about
on her feet. But her hands and arms were still tight and she
held them up in a flexed position when she walked. So she still
looked as if she had significant neurologic problems. This had
a negative impact on any judgment about her other neurologic functions, such as all those difficult to define mental functions. It was hard to describe the subtle changes that were
occurring in her speech and attention. But these changes were
equally, if not more, important in what returning to "normal"
means for everyone. Watching Kara on the BaySide video,
which was made about nine months after her cardiac arrest,
you had trouble understanding some of her speech and you
could see she was easily distracted by little things going on in
the room while they taped. It made you wonder what her inner life was like.

How do we judge someone else's inner life? Mostly, I
think, we assume it is just like our own. And we do this based
on outward appearances. If someone looks and acts like us, he
or she must think like us. When someone moves and reacts in
ways that are different from us we really have no way of knowing, but we often make assumptions that can be far from the
truth. It is common for people to assume the worst about someone with a form of brain damage called choreoathetotic cere-

bral palsy. This is a type of brain injury that occurs in infants and results in a severe movement problem that is something like the movements Kara had early in her hospitalization. If someone with choreoathetotic cerebral palsy achieves walking, they often twist and lurch in a precarious way that is frightening to watch. You are sure a trip or a fall is about to happen with every movement. Their speech is often thick and poorly enunciated, making it difficult to understand them. Thus, for reasons that are obvious we judge that such people have little to say, not just that they say little. This is the subject of Christy Brown's excellent book about himself, *My Left Foot*. His problem of making himself understood is, to a lesser degree, Kara's problem. Her speech is blocked by her problems with control of her movements and her movements look different from what we consider normal. But I don't think her thoughts are any different than any other fifteen-year-old girl's, except that they may be more sensitive and mature.

While Maryann and I were writing this book, we often sent e-mail back and forth. Now and then I wrote directly to Kara. It was a way to judge her inner life that I could not gauge from our short conversations Monday nights driving her home to Bath from a day at BaySide. Maryann keyed in these particular notes as Kara dictated the following e-mail exchange:

FROM: INTERNET...
TO: walter allan...
DATE: 1/9/96

Anyway, I am not the only author in our family.
Here is Kara's story that she dictated to her tutor
Betsy:

Santa asked me, "Now, what would you like for Christmas, Kara Mia?" "I would like a pair of Doc Marten shoes," I said. So his elf came in and said, "Yes, okay, fine." Kara Mia said "Yes." Then she laughed. Kara Mia used to be my imaginary friend. I used to talk to her. We talked about people and toys. We talked about ourselves. Kara Mia stayed home when I went places. If I needed her, she would have come, but I never needed her. Sometimes Kara Mia made me laugh when I was supposed to be serious. She never got me in trouble. I thought it was pretty neat to have her around. It gave me an excuse to talk to myself.

FROM: INTERNET...
TO: kara...
DATE: 1/10/96

Kara,
Ann and I liked what you wrote with Betsy's help about "Kara Mia." Imaginary friends are a great thing, especially when you are young. My brother Mike had an imaginary friend, only it was a HORSE! He would talk to it as he galloped around our yard. Then we (our sister Tish and me) could not hear what he was saying. Whenever our family went anywhere in the car Mike would tie his imaginary horse to the back fender before he got in. When we got to where we were going he would go around to the back of our car and untie his horse and gallop away. We used to make terrible fun of him for this. But Mike did not let that stop him. I am sure the horse did the same for him that Kara Mia did for you.
Dr. Allan or Uncle Walt (take your pick)

FROM: INTERNET...
TO: walter allan...
DATE: 1/10/96

Hi, Uncle Walter!
What was the horse's name? Maybe it was Mr. Ed. Mr. Ed could talk and sing. He could jump four feet and roll around. I think that Mr. Ed was mad at you because you made fun of him. Did you ever have an imaginary friend?
Good-bye. Kara

FROM: INTERNET...
TO: kara...
DATE: 1/11/96

Kara,
That was a funny guess for my brother Mike's horse, but it
was not Mr. Ed. Your Dad will have to fill you in on who
these characters are, but Mike's imaginary horse was called
Topper. He called him Topper because that was Hopalong
Cassidy's horse's name and Mike just loved Hoppy. He had
Hoppy guns and holsters and a black shirt just like Hoppy
did. I think Mike wanted to be Hopalong Cassidy. It was
terrible of me to make fun of Topper but that's what big
brothers are best at. How about big sisters? Does Guerin
ever make fun of you?
Uncle Walter

FROM: INTERNET...
TO: walter allan...
DATE: 1/11/96

Dear Uncle Walter,
Yes, Guerin did make fun of me. She would tease me and
say, "You are really creepy. Where is Kara Mia right now?
You need to get a life." I would say to her, "You need to get
a life, yourself. Kara Mia is my friend and she is up in the
attic."
Love, Kara

FROM: INTERNET...
TO: kara...
DATE: 1/12/96

Kara,
That was the way to stick up for your imaginary friend.
Saying she was in the attic. Great. I bet Guerin never went
up there to check, did she?
Your Imaginary Uncle, Walter

With Maryann's help, I was getting a glimpse of Kara's
imagination which seemed to be flourishing. But there were

159

more insights to be had, thanks to the e-mail. Just before Maryann gave her grand rounds I wrote Kara a note about the videotape of her sessions with Sue Rhyberg. At dinner the night before Kara did a funny thing which probably reflected upon her short attention span at the time. She was feeding herself a bite of potato with her fork when she decided to have a bite of roll. Leaving her fork in her mouth, she reached down with the same hand, picked up the roll and brought it to her mouth. I happened to be looking right at her when she realized that she still had the fork in her mouth. We both broke out in howls of laughter.

Later at the Anglim's house, Kara watched her hospital speech therapy sessions on the tape Maryann would show at the rounds. She watched intently and laughed when she saw herself lean forward during a quiet moment in the session and say, "Hi, Mom!" into the microphone. I knew she was paying attention and must have reflected upon what she looked like at that point in her recovery as Maryann, Tom, Ann and I did. I wanted to put a positive spin on what she saw and thought. As it turned out she could do this herself.

FROM: INTERNET
TO: kara
DATE: 2/2/96

Dear Kara,
Here is what I thought after I saw the videotape of your speech therapy in May and June...Have you ever seen a really good magician? You know the kind that can make rabbits appear in empty old hats, or birds fly out of empty fish bowls? These really good magicians will talk and talk while they wave their arms around so you do not see the trick and then TA-DUM - there's the rabbit or the bird. And we, in the audience can't really believe what we saw so we say, "How DID you do that?" and want them to do it again so we can see the trick. We don't ever really think it is magic. So, when I saw how you changed from May to June I thought to myself, "How DID you do that?" But then I thought that trick was nothing. How about how you changed from June to last Monday night? You know the night you

tried your famous <eat the food and the fork and then the roll trick>. That was the funniest thing I ever saw at a restaurant. How DID you do that?

Kara replies: "Well, Uncle Walter, first you get some food on your fork and you put it in your mouth but you don't take the fork out and you reach for the roll with the hand you used to put the fork in your mouth and ..." No, not that trick! How DID you do that other trick of getting so much better? If you can remember, I wish you would tell me. Otherwise I AM going to think it is magic.

love, Uncle Imaginary Walter

FROM: INTERNET
TO: walter allan
DATE: 2/3/96

Dear Uncle Walter,
Kara Mia was the one who helped me get better. She helps me by telling me I had to get better. At first I felt that there was nobody like me but now I know that everyone likes me because they are helping me with my healing process. So it is hard work and magic that is getting me better in many ways. Sometimes I feel sad when someone gets sick or dies but mostly I feel happy because there is a good reason because I can tell I'm getting better. I can feel it in my heart.
Love, Kara

When I think about these early e-mail notes from Kara and the other times when she and I talk as much as a fifteen-year-old and a fifty-three-year old doctor and friend can, I think there is no doubt she has a rich inner life. "But will she ever be normal?" you ask. Here is a story I tell in reply:

Ann and I took Kara, Maryann and Tom to walk at Prout's Neck along the ocean on a sunny Saturday in May 1996. It is a four-mile walk and Kara fell twice, one time bruising her knee. She fell because of her still impaired gait, although Maryann jokingly accused Tom and me of pushing her. The next Monday when we showed up at the Anglims with Kara, Tom announced that he was going to show me their newest purchase. "It is a neurologist's dream," he said as he escorted me outside to see a twelve-foot diameter trampoline. I was dumbfounded. Maryann said she had not mentioned it to me because she knew that if she had asked my "professional opinion" about a trampoline for Kara, I would have been against it. "Damn right," I thought. "Do you want to see Kara jump on the trampoline?" Maryann asked. It was drizzling and the trampoline was wet. Kara was all for it, climbing up without help. First she jumped up and down on her knees and then she stood up and, without a thought, jumped over onto her back, laughing all the time. I climbed up and did some silly jumping with her. I could not believe it. After her falls during our walk I was not prepared to see her be so agile on a trampoline. It is surprises like that that make me say, "Normal? Well, you just never know."

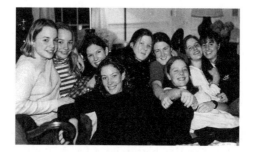

Kara's fifteenth birthday party in March 1996.

CHAPTER 31

Patty and Maryann

❧ ❧ ❧

I was one of those children who loved school. I hated Fridays, loved Mondays and always had my homework done on time and perfectly. I went to a grade school called St. Mary's in a suburb of Chicago named Riverside and I remember so much about it. I remember the red shoes that I wore on the first day of kindergarten; I remember proposing to a boy named Ricky in first grade; I remember getting sent out into the dark hall in second grade by Sr. Donna Marie because I was laughing too much; I remember our class singing with Sr. Patrick Marie through a sudden storm that blackened the sky in third grade and I remember my friend Brigitte laughing so hard at lunch that milk came out of her nose; I remember learning about the Allegheny and the Monongahela Rivers in fourth grade; I remember hating ballroom dance class in fifth grade; I remember the intricate game of tag we developed in sixth grade that constantly had us in trouble for the ultimate infraction: "running on the playground;" I remember puppy love in seventh grade; I remember eighth grade because that was the first time I had a teacher I didn't like. I had a perfect childhood and that is why I remember so much about it. But I also remember my friend Patty died in seventh grade from a brain tumor.

Patty didn't live in my neighborhood, but at school we were good friends. In Catholic school in the fifties, the classes were usually organized by height, the short children sat in the front of the class and the tall children sat in the back. Every time a formal occasion occurred, we were lined up by height for a procession. So, Patty and I became friends because we were the same height. In third grade she sat behind me in class and I remember the teacher coming to her desk during our penmanship period and kindly asking her why her handwriting had become so shaky over the summer. Her answer should have been, "It's because I have a brain tumor, Sister," but, the diagnosis had yet to be made so the answer became, "I will try harder to do better, Sister." After hearing the conversation, I had to look over my shoulder to observe Patty's penmanship for myself. Her writing was legible but each word was filled with tremulous letters. "Hmm," I thought, "those letters are very shaky." I worried that I might get shaky handwriting, too. And then I smiled at Patty and told her that I could still read her handwriting, so there was nothing to worry about.

Soon Patty was gone from our third grade classroom. Of course, now I can look back and know that she was having her brain surgery and months of rehabilitation and months of anguish for her parents. In fourth grade she came back to class, a totally different child than the healthy looking little girl with shaky handwriting that left the year before. She was so frail and delicate. Her fair and freckled skin was now so pale. She wore a little pink bonnet to hide her bald head, shaved for surgery and now left bald by radiation. She used to be one of the smartest in the class; now she was not. She used to be one of the cutest girls; now she was the sickest. She used to be one of my spunkiest classmates; now she was the slowest.

But was it sad and did we pity her? No, because we weren't allowed to look on Patty as sad. We were only allowed to look upon her as a courageous classmate from a courageous family. That was the expectation and that is what we did. Patty wasn't in school much from fifth grade to seventh grade. Every now and then she would come into our class for a few weeks and then she would leave for a few months. In seventh grade she died. Our whole class went to her funeral which I observed with twelve-year-old eyes. I even remember where I sat in the church that morning. I remember the eulogy. I still have the holy card that records her date of birth and date of death. I still have her picture.

The priest who gave the eulogy was the priest who had helped Patty and her family through the entire process of her illness and death. In the eulogy, he related an incident at the very end of Patty's life in which he was praying with her. He asked her to repeat after him as he said, "Dear Jesus, forgive me my sins." Patty repeated instead, "Dear Jesus, I love you." I know why she did that. It was because she was too sweet and innocent to have ever sinned. That was why in the emergency room, when the priest gave Kara the last rites and asked God to forgive Kara her sins, I said, "She hasn't any sins." She couldn't answer, so I did for her.

After eighth grade I went to an all-girls Catholic high school called Nazareth Academy. It was an excellent school where I received a classically-oriented education. My schooling was steeped in Greek and Roman literature and there I learned about many writing tools, one of which was foreshadowing. When I look back on my memories of Patty with my forty-seven-year-old eyes, the word and technique of foreshadowing comes to my mind. There are so many similarities, only now Kara is Patty, I am Patty's mother and the diagnosis has shifted to anoxic brain injury. That family's story foreshadowed my family's story. I can look back and know how her parents felt to have Patty go back to school so differently than she had left it. They must have known that Patty's tumor would eventually kill her, but they struggled to maintain as much normalcy as possible for their daughter. I can imagine how they must have felt having her leave their side after months of being with her in the hospital. I can understand each and every one of their heartaches. I can only guess how difficult it was for them to have all of Patty's healthy classmates at her funeral. I understand their bravery. Watching Patty and her family helped to prepare me for my future, only of course, I didn't know it at the time. Maybe that is why I paid such close attention to the whole process. I am just lucky that I had such good teachers.

When Kara started her second year at the local high school, her teachers asked me to talk to them about Kara's diagnosis, her medical, neurologic and rehabilitative needs, and her emotional state. I carefully prepared a talk that covered each of these topics and at the end I said, "What do I ask of each of you? I ask that you look upon Kara, not with pity but with an understanding of her courage. I ask that you help mend her broken little wings and help her fly again." Now that I think of it, that is what Patty's parents tried to do for her and that is what Patty's parents taught me. I learned so much from my schooling and I am grateful for all that my parents did to educate me at such fine institutions and I am grateful for all of my learned teachers and professors. But, I think that my most important lesson was taught to me by a third grader with shaky handwriting who was the same height as I was.

CHAPTER 32

The Sun and The Wind

 ᷝ ᷝ ᷝ

Recently Tom and I went to a birthday party where the request was that we not bring any presents but that each guest write down the five books that were most influential in our lives. That assignment became a topic of discussion for the weeks preceding the party as we mentally examined our personalities and what books had shaped them. One of the books that appeared upon my list was *Aesop's Fables,* and my favorite fable of his was the one entitled "The Sun and The Wind." In this story the Wind and Sun are arguing over which is the stronger and more powerful. They decide to have a contest to see who will be the winner. They spy on the earth a person with wearing a coat. Whoever can get the coat off the man will be declared the stronger of the two. The Wind goes first. He blows hard and mightily, but the harder he blows, the closer the man holds the coat to his body. The Sun follows with his constant, warm beams and, of course, the man removes his coat. I loved this story when I was a little girl, and I even loved the picture which illustrated this fable in my book. Even as a youngster, I understood the fable's message was an important one.

Now my family will be the first to tell you that I have not perfectly incorporated this fable into my personality. Guerin could tell you about the day that she put the dead snake in the mailbox, and I went ballistic for about a week. Kara could tell you about the day that she thought that she could help decorate the brand new wallpaper by drawing colorful crayon flowers upon it, and again I went ballistic for another week. Tom could tell you about the time he lied to me about not knowing that the children were home early from school.

167

As a result of that lie, he lived with a wife more like the Wind than the Sun for quite a few days. I am sure that they would each willingly add many more stories to these. What I have learned since April 7, 1995, is that none of these things really matter. The snake in the mailbox is now a family joke. I wish I would have never replaced the wallpaper with the crayon flowers drawn upon it; it would have been a piece of Kara's art history. No harm came to the girls that afternoon they were home alone and they probably benefited from their increased responsibility. What I have learned is that the fable is true.

So, I take that fable with me when I need it. This past summer I used it as the time approached for Kara to enter her second year of high school. It was two weeks before school was to have begun and Kara had no program or schedule or aide designated for her. "Hmm...," I thought, "Kara cannot afford to have one wasted day of school. All of the other students have their schedules and that is Kara's right, also." Routines are an important part of Kara's recovery and I also knew that she should be starting her school year with the routine that would set the standard for the entire year. So, I called the appropriate people to set up a meeting where we could collaboratively agree upon the most effective program for Kara's education for 1996-97.

The telephone call to the school office was less than satisfactory because I was told that no meetings with teachers happened in the summer because of the teachers' union contracts. This was a bad omen because it meant that Kara's schedule would not be set until after school began in September. This would mean wasted days for her that had no direction or educational advantage to them. "Hmm...," I thought, "am I the Wind or the Sun?" In other words, "Do I scream or do I overcome them with gentle persuasion?"

Luckily for our family, we are surrounded by the best professionals in the state of Maine. Kara's doctors and therapists are all devoted to her healing process and every victory is felt by them as intensely and joyously as it is felt by Tom and Guerin and me. They are fierce advocates for Kara and they will tolerate nothing less than the optimal treatment for her recovery. They know that I call them my "lobby group" and I knew that I needed them now. Tom and I trust them totally, and we always listen to them. They are the objective balance to our subjective assessments, hopes and goals.

A quick call mobilized my lobby group. A meeting where Kara's BaySide therapists, Dr. Allan, a representative from the high school, Kara's summer tutors and Tom and I all convened immediately to discuss the plan for Kara's second year at high school. With input from all these professionals and the overriding tone of optimism and trust in recovery for Kara, a strong and definite plan was developed. Kara needed an appropriate schedule and a permanent aide from the first day of school. This group arbitrated the perfect balance of academics and therapy for her. They built in enough flexibility for change if the plan needed to be adjusted. Most importantly, the high school staff listened to the advice of the experts and followed through in every detail.

The result was that Kara now has wonderful teachers and classes, and her aide for this second year of high school, Leslie, is fun and smart and the perfect combination of taskmaster and comic. The school year couldn't be going better. Kara's first report card was filled with four As and two Bs and many teachers' comments about hard work and commitment. I remember the day in April 1995 when Kara was a patient in the Special Care Unit and Dr. Bagwell told me about her patient who was as ill as Kara and who came back to visit with a report card filled with good grades. I remember hoping that someday we could do the same. Now we can and the first free day that Kara and I have, we will drive to Portland and visit Dr. Bagwell. We will bring Kara's report card and a bag of candy Sour Patch Kids because that is what Dr. Bagwell told us was one of her favorite things.

Just as Aesop had a lesson with every fable, there is a lesson in this chapter. The lesson is that no family can go through this without the help of their family, friends and the professionals who surround them. The lesson is that strong opinions based in fact and medical knowledge will provide the best care for the person who needs it. The lesson is that the constant and persistent and loving warmth of the Sun will outdo the bravado of the Wind every time.

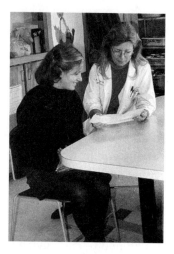

The day comes when Kara can show Dr. Bagwell her all-A report card (except for B's in Gym and chorus).

CHAPTER LAST

Dear Mom...Dear Kara...

છે છે છે

This is not the last chapter in Kara's recovery; it is merely the last chapter in our experiences up to this day. When we were searching for a publisher to handle this manuscript, we knew that we had to find one who dealt with this category of story. But what was the category of our story? Is it a mother's tale? No, it is more than that because it is also told from the physician's point of reference. Is it an article for a medical journal? No, it is more than that because it is also told from the mother's/nurse's point of reference. Is it an explanation of Long QT syndrome? No, it is more than that because there is as much neurology and psychosociology as cardiology in this book. Is this a how-to-book dealing with coping with a tragic illness? No, it is more than that because it is also a documentary steeped with medical facts. Just what type of book is this? The answer to that question is simply that it is a love story. If Kara were to write me a letter, I know just what it would say. It would echo the words of Celine Dion in her song "Because You Loved Me." It would say:

Dear Mom,

You were my strength when I was weak.
You were my voice when I couldn't speak.
You were my eyes when I couldn't see.
You saw the best there was in me.
Lifted me up when I couldn't reach.
You gave me faith because you believed.
I'm everything I am because you loved me.

Love, Kara

And I would think back to those days when Kara was in a coma. And I would think back to those first hours when Kara was on a ventilator in the Special Care Unit. And I would think back to my education at Loyola and the philosophy classes I sat through where we discussed keeping patients alive through "extraordinary means." And I would think back to my nursing classes where I formed my opinions of what "extraordinary means" are. And I would think back to my nursing professors drilling into my head, "You are your patients' advocate." And I would think back to when I saw Dr. Allan as he came to do his initial exam of Kara and I asked him, "Will you help us?" And I would think back to how he looked me clearly in the eye and said, "Yes."

What I was really asking him was a reflection of all of the medical ethics and philosophy and theology I had learned through my many years of Catholic education. Just as most other students at Loyola University in Chicago, I had taken my required theology and philosophy courses because I had to take them to graduate and just as most other Loyola students, I quickly came to enjoy and learn from them. I sat and listened to many discourses on the soul and morality and from these classes and discussions formed my personal philosophy of ethics and morals and right and wrong. The gift which I received from Loyola was that I was forced to face these issues and develop a philosophy before I actually needed one. What I was really asking Dr. Allan was, "If her life can only be sustained by extraordinary means, will you help us let her die? If we just need extraordinary means to get her over this critical period, will you help us let her live?"

For our family, the decision was easy because Kara did have brain waves on the EEG that was done a few hours after her admission to Maine Medical Center. But there was an even bigger sign than that. Kara collapsed on a Friday and on Monday I asked her to smile for me and I saw that same mischievous grin that was Kara through and through. I knew then that Kara was herself inside that sick and frail little body and that I would be her strength and voice and eyes until she had them back again on her own.

Many months after Kara had been discharged from the hospital, I asked Dr. Allan if he knew what I meant that night in the Special Care Unit when I asked him if he would help us. "Yes," he said, "I knew." "Well," I replied, "I had a clear sense of our options with Kara because I had studied and thought so much about it because of my Catholicism. But you aren't Catholic. How did you figure it all out?" "Oh, years of experience with these decisions, Maryann, made me see clearly what you were facing," he answered.

Kara's progress is in an ever-evolving state and as I write this, she is still a handicapped child, but every day less so than the day before. It is winter of 1996 now as I write this but my summer worry was that Kara would have a boring summer. She still depends upon us for projects and entertainment and I feared that the summer would be long and dull for her. But that fear was unfounded. She went to rehab in Portland three days per week and the other four days were filled with the Atlantic Ocean and swimming, lobstering, sailing, walking the beach and tubing, and quite a few Sea Dog's baseball games. Academically she was tutored ten hours per week and her cognitive skills are returning at varying rates. Verbally, she is way above her age level while her math is at approximately a sixth-grade level. She can read and understand every word that is shown to her, but reading a book is still hard for her because her eyes do not track as well as they should. But these skills show marked improvement each time Kara is tested and it is easy to be optimistic. Kara's short term memory was damaged by her anoxic brain injury and there was quite a while when she couldn't tell you the day or the date or the month. But this problem, too, slowly improves. Her attention span and ability to focus on a task were affected by the anoxia, but a daily dose of a medication called Cylert has helped this problem. Physically, her gait is still abnormal but regular work with her therapists and the treadmill have helped her walking to become faster and more steady. Her hands still do not work smoothly, but she has progressed to the point where she can use the computer and work zippers. Buttons are still a little hard for her.

Emotionally she is remarkably stable and determined to get better. But do we have days that are tough? Yes, both Kara and I do. For me one of those days came in December, 1996 and I wrote this journal entry that day:

Slow and Steady
Wins the Race

It is December and Kara has completed her first year and a half of high school. Kara reentered school in October, 1995 and her goals that year were not really academic but increasing her endurance, regaining her ability to focus amidst a myriad of distractions and the reentry into social settings. I didn't realize that those were her goals when she started. I thought her goals would be more to do with measurable learning—math and reading and writing. I had to readjust my paradigms, something at which I have become an expert. It was heartbreaking when I realized that my goals for her would not and could not become her goals for the year. But I looked forward with hope to September and her sophomore year and, as a friend reminded me, "Slow and steady wins the race."

It is late winter and the telephone rarely rings for Kara. Her friends eagerly visited her in the hospital but for a long time after that, none came to call or visit. I used to make excuses for them and say things such as, "Oh, they would come but they are too busy with school and soccer and swimming." But I knew the truth and that is that Kara was too slow for them. She looked and acted too differently from them. I was not angry because I understood, although it was still a heartbreak for me. But I have recently realized something. Just as our family had to cry through our losses and readjust to a new Kara, so did her friends. They had to work through their own adolescent mourning period. Much to their credit, they are realizing that she is still the sweet and fun-loving friend that she always was; she is just packaged a little differently now. So, thank you, Kate, for taking Kara for ice cream and watching *Beverly Hills 90210* with her. Thank you, Naomi and Carrie, for taking her in your boat to Holbrooks for lunch. Thank you for saying, "Next week we are going to take Kara to the beach and find her a boyfriend!" Thank you, Amy, for all the sailing adventures that you had with Kara. Thank you, Molly, for all the lunchtimes you spend with Kara. Thank you, Emily and Julia, for driving Kara to school this sophomore year. Thank you, Laurel, for being so watchful over Kara during the Christmas choral concert. You were like her little guardian angel. Thank you, Kate and Georgie, for taking Kara to the Christmas dance at school. There is also a small group of older girls who have consistently taken Kara places and they, along with Kara's peers, seem to know that "Slow and steady wins the race" and aren't embarrassed to be with someone who is slow and not too steady on her feet.

It is time for me to be out in public but I find myself withdrawn into a small group of friends who know what it is like to be me now. That way I can avoid those conversations that are spontaneous and from the heart but leave me heartbroken. I don't have to hear people say, "I'm glad that I'm not you" or "I didn't expect Kara to be so debilitated." Sometimes it feels as if people are making a special effort to be hurtful. Why can't they understand that what I want to hear is "Slow and steady wins the race"?

In June it was time for graduation and as I watched the senior class so wide-eyed and full of wonder at their future, I wondered if Kara would ever graduate with a meaningful diploma. "Slow and steady wins the race, Maryann," I tell myself. "Just trust in the future and work hard helping Kara regain her skills. Don't think. Just be slow and steady." Gradually Kara will find her niche, but in the meantime, I wonder, how many heartbreaks will I have before my heart just gives up and breaks forever? Some days it is hard to be steady and brave and mature and gracious. Some days I just want to run away and never come back. I wonder about my future, too. But what I wonder is if I will ever have another day in my life that isn't laced with sadness and if ever another day will pass that doesn't have a heartbreak in it.

So now you know my dark side. But what I have learned is that it is acceptable to have a sad day and to let the tears flow. What I have also learned is that a sad day is contagious and before you know it, everyone around you will also be having a sad day and all positive and forward progress and fun will stop. So, I allow myself to have such a day every now and then. I say to myself, "Today I am just going to feel sorry for myself and our situation and tomorrow I will be better and face the world with courage and humor." The plain truth is that there is no magic pill or potion to help; strength and determination come from within one's heart and it is a full-time job for me to keep myself strong. It is just that some days I am better at it than others.

And how does Kara fare emotionally? Luckily, she has been given a wonderful sense of humor and she has the ability to laugh at herself. One day, Tom and Kara went to work out on the treadmills at the YMCA. They each were on their own treadmill and Tom ran on his for thirty minutes while Kara walked on hers for the same thirty minutes. After they had finished their workouts, Tom said, "Whew, I am pooped, Kara. How about you?" She answered back to him with her droll smile, "I should be; I'm the one with the cardiac condition." I am amazed at how humbly she asks for and accepts help for tasks which were once so easy for her, tying her shoes, opening heavy doors, cutting her food. In many ways, she is my role model and I find myself saying, "If Kara isn't discouraged, how can you possibly consider being discouraged?" Certainly the hardest thing for her was the loss of her friends and that is what she would verbalize as her saddest problem. "I have no friends, now," she would say, "because I am not cool enough for anyone." One night she said to me, "It has been a year now that this has been going on with me. I wish that my friends could feel what this is like for me because then they would know." That night Tom and I went to bed in tears, moved both by Kara's perception as well as her own sadness.

Every now and then, Walter Allan will e-mail me some of his thoughts about Kara and these are usually reflections of something he observed when our families were together. This e-mail was particularly poignant because it is so true and obvious to those who take the time to notice and reflect:

FROM: INTERNET...
TO: maryann...
DATE: 6/24/96

Maryann,
...and as far as her being gracious and forgiving...who could
doubt that she is all of that and more by the way she greets
each day and all of her ups and downs. I was watching her
handle her spoon while eating her root beer float. She puts
the spoon in her mouth and then gets the correct grip to
dig out the ice cream so it won't fall off of her spoon. Problem solving. And even though she spilled the drink shortly
thereafter—no tears, no throwing the (bad word) spoon and
no cursing her inabilities. The kid's a trooper.
Walt

That is the essence of Kara's personality, and I would hope so
hard that her peers would notice that and accept her as she
now is.

But my biggest and most recurring message to Kara is,
"We can't look at what isn't there. We can only look at what is
there." And what is there is the fact that there is a small group
of young adults who do take Kara to the movies and who do
take her shopping at The GAP and who do take her tubing and
to the beach. What is there are the friends who take her to the
school dances and the basketball games. What is there is that
some perceptive peers are passing into a stage of wonderful
camaraderie with Kara. What is there is the weekly manicure,
pedicure and hair-do by my friend Paula at her beauty shop.
What is there is that we have a small cluster of friends who
help us emotionally and physically. What is there is that Kara
is getting better each day and that I have no doubt that someday she will have an independent and productive life.

This is not just the story of our family, but of many
families helping us to heal Kara. It is the story of her resolute
courage and determination, and it is the story of our faith in
and hope for a complete recovery. It is a story of hard work,
filled with both humor and tears. It is the most important responsibility that I will ever have and I am grateful that I have

the strength of others upon which to draw. It isn't distressing that "Et in Arcadia Ego" because what I have learned is that "Though I walk through the valley of death, I shall fear no evil." With the strength and help of my friends and family and with the attitudes formed by my experiences and education, I can look anyone or anything directly in the eye and not be afraid.

The summer before Kara suffered her cardiac arrest was the summer between her seventh and eighth grade years at school. Kara had been a busy babysitter, popular with both the parents and the children. I always thought that Kara would be a kindergarten teacher when she grows up because she loves children so much. But that summer, she had been offered a spectacular job for two weeks as a mother's helper for an unusual family.

This family consists of a mother who is a psychiatrist and her six children. I called them "The Rainbow Family" because five of the six children were adopted and they ranged in color from white to black with every shade in between. Normally, they had a nanny who helped with the day-to-day family routines, but during this two week vacation at the beach, the nanny was also on vacation and Kara was hired as the mother's helper. Kara loved this family. She loved the mother, Kate, and she loved each of the children. She always told me that when she grew up, she was going to have a family exactly the same as Kate's.

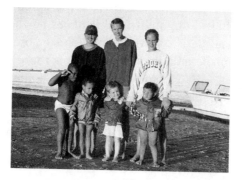

Two-thirds of the "Rainbow Family" with Sarah, Margie and Kara the summer before her arrest.

178

And then Kara collapsed. And then we realized that she had Long QT syndrome. And then we realized that it was a genetic problem and that she should never have children. One day, Kara and I were sitting on the sofa together watching a show about babies and I said to her, in a tentative manner, not knowing what response I would receive, "Kara, do you know that you should never have children." "Yes," she said, "I know." "Do you know why?" I asked her. "Yes," she said, "because my defibrillator will hurt them." "No," I said, "it is not because of your defibrillator. It is because they will inherit the same heart problem that you have. Does that make you feel bad?" "No," she said with her sweet smile, "I will just have a family the same as Kate's." So, that is the final story I will leave with you. That is the story that will tell you that we are all going to be just fine.

And so my letter to Kara will also echo the words of Celine Dion from her song "Fly." It will say simply:

Dear Kara,

Fly, fly, Little Wing
Fly beyond imagining

Love, Mom

↩ ↩ ↩

❧ ❧ ❧

Epilogue
by Father John Powell, S.J.

❧ ❧ ❧

When Maryann Anglim, my sister's niece and also a former theology student of mine, first asked me to write an epilogue to this manuscript, I immediately said, "Yes, of course." Then I received and read the manuscript. I began to get some inkling of what Tom and Maryann and Guerin had been through. My own "Yes, of course" began to look more formidable. Of course, I am honored to put my name in any way on such a manuscript.

Whenever I see or am told about raw human suffering, I usually ask myself: "What if God asked that of me? Could I take it?" I am forced to confess that I do not know. Only God knows the agonies and suffering of the Anglim family.

A doctor named Paul Brand recently published a work called *The Gift Nobody Wants*. This doctor sees suffering—as difficult as it is—as a gift that encourages self-observation. We realign our values in such moments. The Anglims were forced to face the ethical value concerning the sanctity of life in which they knew it would be better to have a somewhat limited Kara than only memories of Kara.

I used to know a man who in his thirties had a heart attack and cancer. The cancer was in his sinuses, so he had to wear a prosthetic false nose. For fear of going out he liked to stay at home and play cards. One day I asked him directly about his suffering. He replied in a matter-of-fact way:

These are the cards God has lovingly dealt me, and these are the cards I will lovingly play.

The last thing he did was wink at me through the oxygen mask as he was whisked to the hospital with a final and fatal heart attack.

I can only admire people like this, like the Anglims, at a distance. I would like to keep "Kara Mia's" picture on the wall of my office, so my own "cards" will always be kept in proportion. What a precious gift Kara is!

John Powell, S.J.
Loyola University of Chicago

❧ ❧ ❧

◆◆◆

Glossary

◆◆◆

Ablated—removed

Agonal complex—a cardiac rhythm that is electrical only and in which the heart does not pump any blood

Ambu bag—a medical device used to force oxygen into an unconscious person's lungs

Anoxia—decreased amount of oxygen in the tissues and organs of the body (see hypoxia)

Anoxic coma—coma resulting from lack of oxygen to the brain

Anoxic injury—injury resulting from lack of oxygen

Arterial line—a plastic catheter which is placed in an artery to provide continual blood pressure readings

Anterior horn cells—cells in the spinal cord that send fibers to the muscles

Arrhythmia—an irregular heart beat

Ascitic belly—accumulation of fluid in the abdominal cavity

Atenolol—a beta-blocking drug

Atrophic—wasting of muscles, tissues, organs or the entire body

Atropine—an antiarrhythmic drug which speeds up the heart rate

Autosomal dominant inheritance—inheritance of trait on one of the non-sex chromosomes and transmitted to everyone who receives the gene. The chance of a child receiving an autosomal dominant gene from an affected parent is fifty percent.

Basal ganglia—deep portions of the brain that control movement quality

Beta-blockers—a group of drugs which are often used to decrease heart rate and blood pressure

Blood gas—a test which reflects the amount of oxygen, carbon dioxide and the acidity/alkalinity of the blood

Bolus—a large amount of fluid given intravenously quickly

Bradycardia—a slow heart rate, usually defined as less than sixty beats per minute

Brain waves—electrical activity from the brain recorded by the EEG

Brainstem—portion of the brain that connects the cerebral hemispheres to the spinal cord and contains the nerves to the head and neck

Brainstem reflex—reflex that involves nerves that originate in the brainstem

Capacitor—a device which stores a charge of electricity

Cardiac catheterization—a procedure in which a catheter is passed into the heart via a vein or artery for diagnosis and treatment of various heart cardiac conditions

Central venous pressure—a measurement of the fluid pressure of a patient by means of tube placed in a blood vessel near the heart which helps in assessing the fluid replacement rate
Choreoathetotic CP—a type of cerebral palsy (CP) that consists of writhing face and limb movements giving the appearance of spastic dancing
Clavicular area—area around the collarbone
Complex partial seizures—seizures consisting of confusion and unusual automatic movements, such as chewing and fumbling with objects
Corneal reflex—reflex consisting of touching the eye over the iris with cotton and watching for the eyelid to quickly close
Coronal images—images in the coronal plane of the brain; as if looking directly through someone's face
Cortex—the portion of the brain that contains the gray matter or the cell bodies of the neurons or nerve cells
Cortical stimulation—process of electrically probing the cortex to identify its function. Stimulation of the cortex in the temporal lobes can evoke memories, speech and complex movements.
Coxsackie virus—a specific virus that can infect the brain and spinal cord simulating polio
Countershocked—defibrillated
Cranial ultrasound scan—computer-generated images of the brain using ultrasound usually performed through the open soft spot in an infant's skull
Cylert—a medication which falls in the category of cerebral stimulants and is used for attention deficit disorder

Defibrillate—to apply an electric shock that stops ventricular fibrillation and hopefully restores the normal beat
Defibrillator—device which can deliver a shock strong enough to change ventricular fibrillation into a normal cardiac rhythm (see ICD)
Diaphragm—the musculomembranous partition between the abdominal and the chest cavities
Diastolic blood pressure—the second number of the blood pressure reading which represents the relaxation phase of the heart
DNA mapping—process of locating the segment of deoxyribonucleic acid (DNA) on a chromosome that is responsible for an inherited trait. Also called "gene mapping."
Dopamine—an emergency drug which is used to increase cardiac output and blood pressure and increase blood flow to vital organs
Dystonia—abnormal movement and tone of the muscles. The tone is usually rigid or spastic in quality and the movements include choreoathetosis and opisthotonus.

ECG—see electrocardiogram
Echocardiogram—an ultrasonic picture of the heart which shows structure as well as motion
EEG—see electroencephalogram
Electrocardiogram—the electrical tracing of the heart's rhythm, consisting of P, Q, R, S, T and U waves.
Electroencephalogram—also known as a brain wave test. It records the very low voltage electrical activity from the cortical neurons by the use of sensitive amplifiers.

Electrophysiology—the study of electrical phenomena as it relates to physical health
EMT—emergency medical technician
Encephalitis—viral infection of the brain
Endotracheal tube—a tube which goes from a patient's mouth or nose into the trachea and allows oxygen to be delivered to the lungs
Epinephrine—an emergency drug, also known as adrenalin, which helps to restore a cardiac rhythm in a cardiac arrest
Esophago-gastro-duodenoscope (EGD)—a flexible and fiberoptic scope which can pass through the mouth, into the esophagus, stomach and upper part of the small intestine
Esophagus—the portion of the digestive tract which goes from the mouth to the stomach
Extensor posturing—act of extending or stretching the arms and legs spontaneously or in response to pinch.
Extubate—the removal of an endotracheal tube from a patient

Flexor movements—movements, mainly of the arms, bending at the elbow
Fluoroscopic—an type of X-ray in which the images are reproduced on a screen for immediate viewing
Frontal sharp wave—a specific finding on EEG in which a sharply contoured brain wave stands out from the other waves coming from the frontal lobe of the brain

Gag reflex—reflex movement of opening the mouth and protruding the tongue after the back of the throat is forcefully touched with a tongue blade
Gastrostomy feeding tube—a tube which goes through the skin of the abdomen into the stomach through which liquid nutritional supplements are given
Gauge—size
Generalized slowing of the EEG—a brain wave pattern that suggests general brain dysfunction that is often seen in coma

Hemisphere, cerebral—one of the two nearly identical halves of the brain above the brainstem
Hippocampus—portion of the brain located in the temporal lobes involved with memory, emotions and sexual drives
Hypotension—subnormal blood pressure
Hypoxia—decreased amount of oxygen in the tissues and organs of the body (see anoxia)

ICD—see implantable cardiac defibrillator
Implantable cardiac defibrillator—an implantable battery-operated, computerized electronic device that acts as a pacemaker for the heart if the rate falls below a preset limit and can sense ventricular fibrillation and defibrillate automatically
Inflammatory response—the response of the human body to injury that eventually leads to repair and healing
Insula—portion of cerebral cortex lying deep in the fissure between the

temporal and frontal lobe of each hemisphere. Its function is poorly understood but it can be associated with speech problems.

Intravenous catheter—a tube placed in a vein through which fluids and medications may be given

Intubate—the insertion of an endotracheal tube into a patient

Invasive monitor—any device placed within the body used for assessing the patient's condition

Ion channels—pores in the membrane of muscle and nerve cells that allow rapid movement of ions across the membrane. The opening and closing of ion channels produce the electrical changes in the membrane that are responsible for muscle contraction and nerve impulse conduction.

IV—see intravenous catheter

Joule—a unit of energy

Lead—an electrode placed upon or in a patient's body to detect electrical activity

Magnetic resonance imaging—a brain scan obtained in a strong magnetic field that produces images in multiple planes of very high resolution

MRI scan—see magnetic resonance imaging

Nasogastric tube—a tube which extends from the stomach through the nose which helps to prevent vomiting as well as serving as a means for nutritional supplements

Neuronal cell death—the loss of neurons from various causes such as anoxia. The biochemical process by which neurons die is an area of intense scientific study.

Neurons—the cells that are responsible for brain electrical activity. Their processes connect the multiple areas of the brain together as well as send impulses to the brainstem and the spinal cord and hence out to the body's muscles and nerves.

Opisthotonus—the involuntary act of bending the head backward at a severe angle while extending the arms and legs. This posture is assumed spontaneously after injuries to the upper brainstem.

Oximeter—a machine which measures the percent of oxygen in the body by means of a probe which is usually placed on a finger

Oxygen saturation—this is represented by a number provided by an oximeter and it measures how well a patient is breathing. A normal, healthy person should have an oxygen saturation of ninety-eight to one hundred percent.

Pace—the action of the implanted pacemaker device which electrically stimulates the heart to beat

Pacemaker—the implantable device which electrically stimulates the heart to beat when the patient's own heart rate falls below a certain preset number

Parsimonious—frugal to excess; stingy; miserly; penurious

PEG—acronym for percutaneous gastrostomy tube
PET scan—see positron emission tomography
Percutaneous—through the skin
Percutaneous gastrostomy tube—see gastrostomy feeding tube
Positron emission tomography—a brain scan obtained using special radioactive isotopes that emit positrons. Because the isotopes are chemicals utilized by the brain, the scans can show brain function as well as anatomy.
Pharynx—the throat
Phrenic nerve—the nerve which stimulates the diaphragm to move
Posturing—involuntary positioning of the limbs
Pulmonary edema—an accumulation of excess fluids in the lungs
Pump—a mechanical device which can be programmed to allow a predetermined amount of fluid to be administered, either through an IV or a feeding tube
Pupillary response—a reflex usually elicited by shining light on the eye and watching for constriction of the pupil

Reactive pupils—pupils that have a normal response to light
Repolarize—an electrical event which recharges the cell membrane or fiber and permits it to fire again
Respirator—a machine which connects to an endotracheal tube and breathes for a patient who is either unconscious or paralyzed (see ventilator; see endotracheal tube)

Sarcophagus—a stone coffin
SCU—see Special Care Unit
Secondary generalization—seizures that begin in one part of the brain and then spread to involve the entire brain are said to secondarily generalize
Secondary seizures—seizures that are produced by some general body dysfunction that reduces blood or glucose delivery to the brain
Sinus Rhythm—a heart rhythm which electrically originates from the sinoatrial node, which is what normally occurs in the heart
Special Care Unit—also known as an Intensive Care Unit
Step-Down Cardiac Unit—the hospital unit to which cardiac patients go after they are past the critical phase of their hospitalization
Sternum—breast bone
Subclavian vein—a vein which has an access near the collarbone
Substantia nigra—an area of the brainstem that contains a dark pigment and is a major part of the extrapyramidal motor system. Dysfunction of this structure produces dystonia that is mainly manifested by decreased movements and increased tone in the muscles. It is the structure that degenerates in Parkinsonism.
Sudden death—an all-inclusive term used to describe any of a number of cardiac diagnoses which strike without warning and carry a high rate of mortality
Supraventricular ectopic pacer—an inappropriate and abnormal pacing focus of the heart which can cause abnormal heart rhythms
Systolic blood pressure—the first number of the blood pressure reading which represents the contraction phase of the heart

Tachyarrhythmia—a heart rate of over one hundred beats per minute with either a regular or irregular rhythm

Tegretol—an anticonvulsant medication

Telemetry—the transmission of a patient's electrocardiographic tracings to a central location where they are watched by skilled personnel

Temperature probe—a device which measures a patient's body temperature

Temporal lobe—the portion of the brain that contains the hippocampus and is important in memory and emotions. The left temporal lobe is very important for language.

Thoracotomy—surgical opening of the chest cavity

Torsion dystonia—an inherited, slowly progressive disease that produces severe rigidity and extensor posturing of the trunk and limbs

Trachea—the windpipe

Tracheostomy—the surgical formation of a hole in the neck into the windpipe to assist breathing

Tracings—the lines on the monitors which denote the patient's condition

Treadmill study—the cardiac information obtained from an ECG during a workout on the treadmill

Triple lumen catheter—a tube with three smaller tubes within it that is inserted into a blood vessel for the administration of fluids, medication or blood

Tripolar lead—a wire with three electrodes that connects the ICD to the heart muscle (see ICD, see lead)

U wave—the ECG wave that appears after the T wave

Vena cava—large vein which carries blood directly back into the heart

Ventilator—a machine which connects to an endotracheal tube and breathes for a patient who is either unconscious or paralyzed (see respirator, see endotracheal tube)

Ventricles—the heart's two chambers of which the right pumps blood to the lungs and the left pumps blood into the aorta

Bibliography

ⴲ ⴲ ⴲ

CHAPTER 2- Shocks:
The management of cardiac arrest and the outcome of out-of-hospital cardiac arrest in situations like Kara's are reviewed in the following chapter:

> Myerburg RJ, Castellanos A: Chapter 26. "Cardiac arrest and sudden cardiac death." In Braunwald E, editor, *Heart Disease: A Textbook of Cardiovascular Medicine* 1992, Fourth edition, W.B. Saunders Co. Philadelphia.

CHAPTER 5- A Doctor's Impressions:
The best clinical information available for predicting outcome in patients with coma lasting at least six hours following cardiac arrest, is found in:

> Levy DE, Caronna JJ, Singer BH, Lapinski RH, Frydman H, Plum F: Predicting outcome from hypoxic-ischemic coma. JAMA 1985;253:1420-1426.

CHAPTER 10- Kara's Medical History:
This report was part of the information I subsequently found in learning about Long QT syndrome. It reviews the neurologic literature of individuals with stories similar to Kara's:

> Pacia SV, Devinsky O, Luciano DJ, Vazquez B: The prolonged QT syndrome presenting as epilepsy: a report of two cases and literature review. Neurology 1994;44:1408-1410.

CHAPTER 12- Long QT Syndrome:
The remarkable story of the molecular biology of Long QT syndrome is found in the following papers by the group in Utah headed by Drs. Vincent and Keating:

> Vincent GM, Timothy KW, Leppert M, Keating MT: The spectrum of symptoms and QT intervals in carriers of the gene for the long-QT syndrome. N Eng J Med 1992;327:846-852.

> Towbin J: Clinical implications of basic research: New revelations about the Long-QT Syndrome. N Eng J Med 1995;333:384-385.

> Curran ME, Splawski I, Timothy KW, Vincent GM, Green ED, Keating MT: A molecular basis of cardiac arrhythmia: HERG mutations cause long QT syndrome. Cell 1995;80:795-803.

Wang Q, Shen J, Splawski I, Atkinson D, Li Z, Robinson JL, Moss AJ, Towbin JL, Keating MT: SCN5A mutations associated with an inherited cardiac arrhythmia, long QT syndrome. Cell 1995;80:805-811

Sanguinetti MC, Jiang C, Curran ME, Keating MT: A mechanistic link between an inherited arrhythmia and an acquired cardiac arrhythmia: HERG encodes the I/Kr potassium channel. Cell 1995;81:299-307.

Wang Q, Curran ME, Splawski I, Burn TC, Millholland JM, VanRaay TJ, Shen J, Timothy KW, Vincent GM, de Jager T, Schwartz PJ, Towbin J, Moss AJ, Atkinson DL, Landes GM, Connors TD, Keating MT: Positional cloning of a novel potassium channel gene: KVLQT1 mutations cause cardiac arrhythmias. Nature Genetics 1996;12:17-23.

The story of Dr. Vincent's discovery of the large kindred with Long QT syndrome in Utah and his efforts on behalf of all patients with this diagnosis is described in the following:

"Michael Vincent's Good Cause" by Peter Michelmore, *Reader's Digest* June 1996, pp 157-162.

The address for the foundation that has helped support families with Long QT syndrome and disseminate information about the condition is:

Sudden Arrhythmia Death Syndrome (SADS) Foundation 540 Arapeen Drive, Suite 207, Salt Lake City, UT 84108.

CHAPTER 13- Kara's MRI:
A paper describing the findings on MRI scan following cardiac arrest similar to those seen in Kara is referenced here:

Fujioka M, Okuchi K, Sakaki T, Hiramatsu K-I, Miyamoto S, Iwasaki S: Specific changes in human brain following reperfusion after cardiac arrest.

CHAPTER 16- Kara's Defibrillator:
A description of internal cardioverter defibrillators is contained in the following chapter. As with all technology, the devices have changed rapidly in the past decade and the description of devices in this chapter covers the newest types. The third generation ICD that was implanted in Kara features computer interrogation of the ICD permitting retrieval of any events so that changes in therapy can be based on actual electrical facts about the event.

Cannom DS: Chapter 29.3 "Internal Cardioverter Defibrillator: Newer Technology and Newer Devices." In Podrid PJ and Kowey PR, editors, *Cardiac Arrhythmia: Mechanisms, Diagnosis and Management* 1995, Williams & Wilkins.

CHAPTER 18- Managed Care?
Katie Beckett's story is partially told by her mother, Julianne, in the following brochure:

> Julianne Beckett, "Comprehensive Care for Medically Vulnerable Infants and Toddlers: A Parents Perspective." In *Equals in this Partnership* 1984, brochure from the National Center for Clinical Infant Programs (Telephone: 703-528-4300)

A source of information about funding for families with children who face prolonged illnesses or recovery are listed below:

> Lynn Robinson Rosenfeld, *Your Child and Health Care. A "Dollars & Sense" Guide for Families with Special Needs* 1994, Paul H. Brookes Publishing Co. Baltimore, MD.

CHAPTER 24- Et in Arcadia Ego:
A discussion of paintings that illustrated Virgil's concept of death even in paradise and the difficulty painters had with this concept is contained the book listed below.

> Erwin Panofsky, "Et in Arcadia Ego: Poussin and the Elegiac Tradition." In *Meaning in the Visual Arts* 1955, Doubleday.

Ian Finlay's garden is described in the article.

> Prudence Carlson, "The Garden on the Hill." *Arts Magazine*, February 1990, p.40.

CHAPTER 26- Changes:
This book, dealing with the evolving nature of the relationship between professionals and families, suggests that what happened between the Anglims and Dr. Allan is possible in other situations:

> Patricia Taner Leff and Elaine H. Walizer, *Building the Healing Partnership. Parents, Professionals and Children with Chronic Illnesses and Disabilities* 1992, Brookline Books, Cambridge, MA.

CHAPTER 27- A Thousand Cranes:
This is the book that tells the story of a Japanese girl with leukemia and the Japanese custom of "senbazuru":

> Eleanor Coerr, *Sadako and The Thousand Cranes* 1990, Dell, New York.

CHAPTER 29- What Does It Mean to have a Gene?:
A review of the latest information about the Long QT syndrome genes is found in:

> Roden DM, Lazzara R, Rosen M, Schwartz PJ, Towbin J, Vincent GM; for the SADS Foundation Task Force on LQTS: Multiple mechanisms in the Long QT syndrome: current knowledge, gaps and future directions. Circulation 1996;94:1996-2012.

CHAPTER 30- "So How is Kara Doing, Dr. Allan?":
An interesting review article of the mechanisms of neurologic recovery following brain ischemic injury is listed along with articles about the

function of the insula and the impact of its injury on speech and language.

Lee RG, van Donkelaar P: Mechanisms underlying functional recovery following stroke. Can J Neurol Sci 1995;22:257-263.

Shuren J: Insula and aphasia. J Neurol 1993;240:216-218.

Habib M, Daquin G, Milandre L, Royere ML, Rey M, Lanteri A, Salamon G, Khalil R: Mutism and auditory agnosia due to bilateral insular damage— role of the insula in human communication. Neuropsychologia 1995;33:327-339.

To order more copies of

Kara Mia

**the story of sudden loss and slow recovery
in a teenager with Long QT syndrome**

ISBN 0-9656501-0-3

<u>By mail</u>
please send your requests to
Seahorse Press
P.O. Box 38
Bath, Maine 04530-1617

Enclose a check for $15.95
$12.95 per book
$3.00 shipping & handling
(Maine residents add $.78 tax)

<u>By phone</u>
call toll-free: **1-888-442-7445**

<u>By fax</u>
call **1-207-442-7445**
Be sure to record your name, address with zip code,
phone number, as well as your Visa or Mastercard
number with expiration date

You may reach us through the Seahorse Press web site:

WWW.gwi.net/SeahorsePress